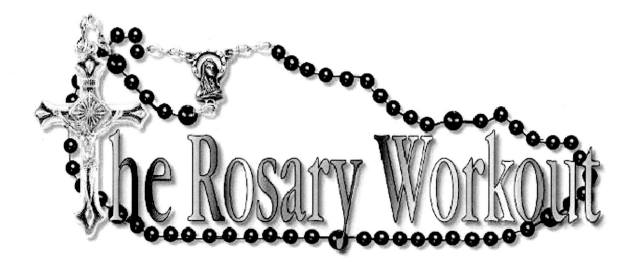

The Rosary Workout

Peggy Bowes

Published by
Bezalel Books
Box 300427
Waterford, MI 48330

www.BezalelBooks.com

Scripture texts in this work are taken from the *New American Bible with Revised New Testament and Revised Psalms* © 1991, 1986, 1970 Confraternity of Christian Doctrine, Washington, D.C. and are used by permission of the copyright owner. All Rights Reserved. No part of the *New American Bible* may be reproduced in any form without permission in writing from the copyright owner.

Excerpts from the English translation of the *Catechism of the Catholic Church* for use in the United States of America Copyright 1994, United States Catholic Conference, Inc. -- Libreria Editrice Vaticana. Used with Permission.

Excerpts from *The Rosary: "The Little Summa"* and *The Catholic Ideal: Exercise and Sports* by Robert Feeney used with permission from the author. These books are available at www.Ignatius.com

All photographs, charts and graphics are either in the public domain or were purchased by the author.

Rosary Workout, LLC strongly recommends that you consult with your physician before beginning any exercise program. You should be in good physical condition and be able to participate in the exercise.

When participating in any exercise or exercise program, there is the possibility of physical injury. If you engage in this exercise or exercise program, you agree that you do so at your own risk, are voluntarily participating in these activities, assume all risk of injury to yourself, and agree to release and discharge Rosary Workout, LLC from any and all claims or causes of action, known or unknown, arising out of Rosary Workout LLC's or the author's negligence.

ISBN 978-0-9823388-6-5
Library of Congress Control Number 2009943356

Send an email to contact@rosaryworkout.com with "Ebook Version" in the subject line to receive a complimentary ebook version of *The Rosary Workout*. The ebook includes additional links and resources as well as color-coded graphics of the workouts. This offer is limited to those who have purchased this book or received it as a gift.

Sign up to receive informative newsletters and updates to *The Rosary Workout* by filling out a contact form at www.rosaryworkout.com/contact.html

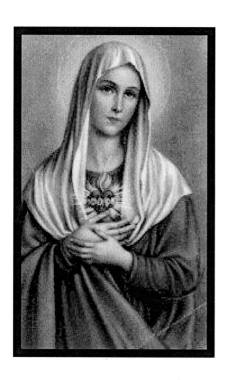

Dedication

This book is dedicated to
the Immaculate Heart of Mary
on her Feast Day,
May 31, 2008,
at Immaculate Heart of Mary Church,
San Antonio, Texas,
birthplace of the author
and her two children.

Sweet heart of Mary, be our salvation.

Praise for
The Rosary Workout

"Anyone who wants to add a spiritual dimension to an exercise routine may find this program to be just what they are looking for. We examined [The Rosary Workout] and it is well written and spiritually enlightening (even if you decide not to exercise).

- CatholicCulture.org review

"I love that Peggy encourages readers to keep a journal that includes not only details about each workout, but also details about spiritual things. Did you go to Confession? Have you been struggling? Do you have a special intention? Tying my physical and spiritual health together in such a tangible way feels right in a way that excites me, that makes me, for once, WANT to work out."

- Sarah Reinhard
snoringscholar.com

"How could I not at least test it out and try it? I could add spiritual growth and renewal at the same time as working toward continued health. I could use the extra prayer time. I could use a new way to lead me into deeper meditation. I could use some guidance from someone who clearly knew fitness. So I tried it. The workout is very well laid out and designed. It can be for the most beginner of beginners, the postpartum mom who is ready to get moving a little more and for those of us in the frigid Midwest it will be wonderful to keep up with in the winter months too. It can be simply implemented with or without exercise equipment (elliptical, recumbent bike, treadmill, etc.) or used just plain old walking or jogging. Pretty versatile and easily accessed. No excuses or limitations."

- Sarah, Catholic blogger
"With a Hopeful Heart"

Foreword

Not long ago I woke up one morning, looked at the note dangling off my bedroom lamp, and made a startling realization - my entire life is organized with post-it notes.

They're everywhere – on the fridge, the bathroom mirror, the coffee table, my recliner, my nightstand, even my breviary.

The problem is that I'm just too busy. I have a hectic job where I wear several hats and have to compartmentalize my day in order to do all of the work that is expected of me. And in between all those tasks, there's the constant flow of e-mail and phone calls. Some days I feel like a broken record, saying over and over again, "Now where was I . . ."

Then there's the family. Although I'm single, I have two elderly parents, six brothers and sisters, seventeen nieces and nephews, a great-niece and two great-nephews – all of whom have their own needs and issues. I also have friends who are in various stages of meltdown as they try to deal with serious illness, addicted spouses, and financial ruin.

And because I have no husband or children to help, everything falls on me - food shopping, paying the bills, cooking, washing the dishes, doing the laundry, emptying the trash, cleaning the litter box and scrubbing toilets.

Besides all this, I have the great privilege of running the perpetual adoration chapel at my parish, which means phone calls coming in at any hour of the day or night – " I can't make my holy hour today" – which means it's time to drop everything and find a sub.

And so I chronicle my life with a daily diary and a 12-pack of post-it notes from Wal-Mart.

It works for me! But I believe it does so because of one very important thing – I indulge myself in nearly three hours of prayer a day.

I can hear you now – three *hours*? Yes! And it's not as hard as you might think. The morning begins with 30 minutes of mental prayer followed by Mass. Every evening I have dinner, watch the news for a few minutes, than slip out to the chapel for a holy hour.

Midway through the day, I need to pray again, to regroup and regain my focus on the Lord. But this is also the perfect time of day to pamper myself with another favorite activity – exercise. As a former fitness instructor, I know exercise is essential for anyone who wants to stay healthy; and as a secular Carmelite, I know prayer is just as essential for anyone who wants to stay holy.

But how does a woman whose entire life is held together by post-it notes find time for both?

Easy. Combine them.

That's what I decided to do one day, combine the Rosary with my regular workout – and it worked so well that I've been doing it ever since.

Depending on the weather and the time of year, I'll either walk at a local track, use an aerobic step, or jog on a treadmill. The exercise always involves mindless repetitions so I can concentrate on the mysteries.

Let me tell you how easy it is to push yourself a little harder while meditating on Jesus carrying that heavy cross up a steep and rocky path to Calvary. How hard can it be to go a bit further considering how far Mary walked – while three months pregnant – to visit Elizabeth? Considering the birth of Jesus, the Transfiguration, the unprecedented miracles of the Incarnation and the Resurrection, makes you feel good in spite of the sweat.

The bottom line is that you *forget the pain* because your mind – and your heart – are elsewhere!

This is why I leaped at the chance to write the foreword for Peggy's book. I've been doing this for years (I thought it was my secret!), which is how I *know* that The Rosary Workout ™ works! It's the answer for anyone who feels they are too time-starved to fit both daily prayer *and* a regular workout into their lives. By combining the two, you not only accomplish both goals, but you give yourself two good reasons to get up and get it done: first, because you need the exercise and second, because if you're like me, it might be the only time of day you'll get to pray the Rosary.

The Rosary Workout ™ is comprehensive and fits people of all fitness and spiritual levels. As a fitness professional and a prayer warrior, Peggy Bowes has employed both of these rare talents to create a plan designed to strengthen both the body and the soul, making this the most complete and essential program on the market today.

Susan Brinkmann, OCDS
Staff Journalist, Editor
Women of Grace ®

Table of Contents

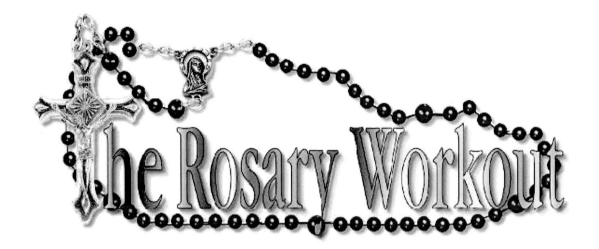

Physical Activity Readiness Questionnaire

1. Before beginning any new exercise program, you should consult your physician, especially if you are pregnant or post-partum, have risk factors for disease, or are recovering from an illness or injury. The PAR-Q form on the next page is a helpful tool to determine any risk factors involved in beginning a new exercise program.

2. If you are exercising and feel any of the symptoms listed below, stop exercising right away:

- Chest pain such as pressure or burning

- Chest pain that goes to the shoulders or down the arm

- Extreme dizziness, feeling of confusion, or weakness

- Extreme shortness of breath or trouble breathing

If any of the symptoms persist, seek medical or emergency assistance right away or call 911.

Physical Activity Readiness Questionnaire (PAR-Q) and You

Regular physical activity is fun and healthy, and increasingly more people are starting to become more active everyday. Being more active is very safe for most people. However, some people should check with their doctor before they start becoming much more physically active.

If you are planning to become much more physically active than you are now, start by answering the seven questions in the box below. If you are between the ages of 15 and 69, the PAR-Q will tell you if you should check with your doctor before you start. If you are over 69 years of age, and you are not used to being very active, check with your doctor.

Common sense is your best guide when you answer these questions.

Please read the questions carefully and answer each one honestly: Check Yes or No

YES	NO		
☐	☐	1.	Has your doctor ever said that you have a heart condition <u>and</u> that you should only do physical activity recommended by a doctor?
☐	☐	2.	Do you feel pain in your chest when you do physical activity?
☐	☐	3.	In the past month, have you had chest pain when you were not doing physical activity?
☐	☐	4.	Do you lose your balance because of dizziness or do you ever lose consciousness?
☐	☐	5.	Do you have a bone or joint problem that could be made worse by a change in your physical activity?
☐	☐	6.	Is your doctor currently prescribing drugs (for example, water pills) for your blood pressure or heart condition?
☐	☐	7.	Do you know of <u>any other reason</u> why you should not do physical activity?

IF YOU ANSWERED

YES to one or more questions

Talk with your doctor by phone or in person BEFORE you start becoming much more physically active or BEFORE you have a fitness appraisal. Tell your doctor about the PAR-Q and which questions you answered YES.
~You may be able to do any activity you want – as long as you start slowly and build up gradually. Or, you may need to restrict your activities to those, which are safe for you. Talk with your doctor about the kinds of activities you wish to participate in and follow his/her advice.
~Find out which community programs are safe and helpful for you.

NO to all questions

If you answered NO honestly to all PAR-Q questions, you can be reasonably sure you can:
~Start becoming much more physically active – begin slowly and build up gradually. This is the safest and easiest way to go.
~Take part in a fitness appraisal -- this is an excellent way to determine your basic fitness so that you can plan the best way for you to live actively.

DELAY BECOMING MUCH MORE ACTIVE:

~If you are not feeling well because of a temporary illness such as a cold or a fever – wait until you feel better; or
~If you are or may be pregnant – talk to your doctor before you start becoming more active.

Please note: If your health changes so that you then answer YES to any of the above questions, tell your fitness or health professional. Ask whether you should change your physical activity plan.

Informed use of the PAR-Q: Reprinted from ACSM's Health/Fitness Facility Standards and Guidelines, 1997 by American College of Sports Medicine.

Preface

I'm very excited about this book as it's the culmination of all I've been studying and practicing during my lifelong dedication to both the Rosary and to regular exercise. My mother taught me to pray the Rosary at a young age, and my family of seven prayed the Rosary together during the frequent travels required of my father's Air Force career. I came to associate the Rosary with family, travel and journeys and found that frequent Rosary recitation helped me to grow spiritually. The more I prayed the Rosary, the more blessings I received.

When I left home to attend the Air Force Academy, I found comfort and relief of my homesickness by silently praying the Rosary during the long marches of Basic Training. I said the Rosary during the stressful Air Force survival training as well as during personal trials. As an Air Force pilot, I even prayed the Rosary on long solo flights. Eventually, I began praying the Rosary while exercising — cycling, running, swimming and on cardio equipment in the gym. I found the rhythm of the exercise cleared my head and actually enhanced my prayer and meditation.

My passion for exercise led me to become certified as a group fitness instructor. I taught aerobics classes and designed motivational fitness programs for the Air Force personnel in my squadron. When I became pregnant, I was fortunate to be assigned as a counselor and fitness coordinator at an Air Force Health and Wellness Center. This was a very eye-opening experience for me. I quickly realized that most people did not share my passion for exercise and regarded it as a chore. They were bewildered and intimidated, and did not know how to exercise properly or effectively. Even people who exercised regularly were confused by all the misinformation spread in the media, the internet and by word of mouth. I found great satisfaction in educating Air Force personnel and their families as to how exercise could be both enjoyable and productive. I was thrilled when someone whom I'd counseled came back later to tell me how exercise had changed his or her life for the better.

I left the Air Force to stay home with my children but continued my education in the field of health and wellness by becoming certified as a personal trainer, SPINNING® instructor and Lifestyle and Weight Management Consultant. I started a business administering fitness and metabolic testing, along with weight loss counseling. By actually measuring the metabolic rate of hundreds of clients, I learned firsthand of the positive effect of regular exercise on metabolism. Almost without exception, all my clients who exercised regularly had a higher measured metabolic rate than predicted for their age, weight and gender. It was very exciting and encouraging to prove that exercise really does pay off!

I also discovered through counseling sessions, that my clients faced many varied obstacles in trying to establish and maintain a habit of regular exercise. I had to draw on experience and education to come up with creative ways to help these reluctant exercisers reach their goals. I enjoyed counseling and working with people, especially when I could make a positive impact on their lives. All these experiences were very rewarding and would ultimately play a significant role in the writing of this book.

When my husband retired from the Air Force, we decided to make a dramatic lifestyle change. We sold our house and nearly all our possessions and bought an RV so that we could travel as a family and homeschool our two children.

I was riding my bike and praying the Rosary on one of our travel stops when I realized that I could apply the Rosary prayers to my planned workout: interval training (short bursts of speed followed by a longer, slower recovery period), which perfectly matched the structure of the Rosary prayers — three short prayers (Glory Be, Fatima Prayer and Our Father), followed by a longer decade of ten Hail Mary's. I came home and started writing, applying the principles of exercise science to a program centered on praying the Rosary.

I did not want my exercise program to be yet another entry on the crowded list of "quick-fix, instant-result" workout plans. Instead, I decided to create a plan that would help a person improve both physically and spiritually. This is not a multi-tasking prayer-and-exercise plan, but rather an integrated approach to taking care of the body and soul together.

In order to be certain that there was not a similar concept published, I searched far and wide and found many Christian exercise programs, but they all tended to be aerobics classes with Christian music. Although I found references to people or groups who prayed the Rosary while exercising, there were no structured workout plans. I finally came across Robert Feeney's book, The Catholic Ideal: Exercise and Sports which introduced me to the idea of the Rosary as "Mary's School". Through the Rosary, Mary leads us closer to her Son, Jesus. The "school" concept applied to my exercise program since I wanted to teach the reader the "how and why" behind my exercise program. Furthermore, Mr. Feeney's explanation of three levels of Mary's "Rosary school" meshed perfectly with my concept of Beginner, Intermediate and Advanced workouts. I therefore adopted the concept of "Mary's school" as the spiritual foundation for The Rosary Workout™.

During my research, I became an enthusiastic student of the Rosary. I began to read and study the Bible as well as countless books, pamphlets and websites on the Rosary. The more I read and studied, the more I began to understand the mysteries of the Rosary and the more material I had at my disposal during my Rosary meditation.

I "field tested" The Rosary Workout™ program as I trained for an Adventure Race and a triathlon. I am very pleased with the results, both physically and spiritually. It is my humble hope that this work will in some way enrich your life here on earth and will aid you in your journey to eternal life. May God bless you in your efforts.

Peggy Bowes

Introduction

Congratulations on your decision to begin The Rosary Workout™, an integrated prayer and exercise program! Although many people pray the Rosary while exercising, this program is unique. It is not "just" exercising while reciting the Rosary. The Rosary Workout™ is structured to present a continual physical and spiritual challenge. I have combined modern exercise science with Rosary prayer to create a series of workouts that are spiritually uplifting, physically challenging and motivational.

What is The Rosary Workout™?

The Rosary Workout™ is a means to care for body and soul together. It is a goal-centered program focused on the integration of exercise, prayer and meditation to work the "muscles of the spirit" in harmony with the muscles of the body.

The *Catechism of the Catholic Church* (*CCC*) teaches that the body and soul are one: *"The unity of the soul and body is so profound that one has to consider the soul to be a "form" of the body."* (*CCC*, Section 365)

We are created in God's image, and we are masterpieces of God's creation. Our human person, body and soul, is a gift from God -- it is of utmost importance to care for both.

The foundation of The Rosary Workout™ is the ability to meditate during exercise. Rhythmic cardiovascular exercise at a moderate pace serves to open the mind to clearer thought and heightened awareness. The Rosary Workout™ uses this physiological response to exercise for a higher purpose, namely directing the clarity of mind toward meditative prayer.

The program builds on this foundation with a scholastic approach to exercise and prayer. I will show you how Mary is our teacher in the "school" of the Rosary, leading us to a deeper understanding and love of her Divine Son and ultimately, our Heavenly Father. Concurrently, I will guide you in a periodized exercise program using the unique structure of the Rosary and the latest principles of exercise science to advance your fitness level and overall physical health.

The ultimate aim of the program is to lead you to become more Christ-like. By reflecting on the mysteries of the Gospels, you will learn to imitate the virtues portrayed in the examples of Jesus and Mary.

The Rosary Workout™ is designed for you!

Every person is at a different point on his or her journey to physical and spiritual health. Some have achieved a high level of physical fitness but are longing for spiritual fulfillment. Others enjoy a rich spiritual life but are stymied as to how to care for their bodies. Still others are somewhere in the middle of the two extremes. Regardless of your current level of physical and spiritual fitness, you will find valuable information and inspiration — The Rosary

Workout™ is structured to benefit everyone. I will teach you how, when and where to begin, allowing you to progress at your own pace, always reaching for a greater level of both physical and spiritual fitness.

Consider the fact that you have a role to play in God's Divine Plan. He has chosen you for a specific mission and has bestowed upon you the gifts and graces to accomplish it. By enriching and improving your physical and spiritual health, you can best achieve your unique purpose on earth. The Rosary Workout™ is designed to equip you physically and spiritually for the challenges that lie ahead.

If you are not familiar with the Rosary, please refer to the Appendix for a tutorial on how to pray the Rosary and a list of the prayers and mysteries. Don't lose heart if you are not accustomed to praying the Rosary or if you find Rosary meditation challenging. As Sister Lucia of Fatima says, *"Even for those souls who pray without meditating, the simple act of taking the beads in hand to pray is already a remembrance of God, of the supernatural."* Although the Rosary is considered a Catholic prayer, people of other faiths are drawn to its simple beauty. The Rosary predates the Reformation and is a Biblical prayer -- its origin and prayers are rooted in Sacred Scripture.

To the best of my knowledge, all references to religious websites provided in this book reflect orthodox Catholic teaching faithful to the Magisterium of the Church. By providing a link, I in no way imply that I (and more importantly the Church) agree with everything you might find on the rest of that site, or any links it in turn provides. I have checked all my religious links at Catholic Culture's website, a site that reviews other Catholic websites. Since many websites that claim to be "Catholic" do not follow Church teachings, I rely on Catholic Culture to help me determine whether a given site is faithful to the Magisterium: **www.CatholicCulture.org/reviews**

The Rosary Workout™ is a physical and spiritual program which is not intended to be used with non-Catholic or non-traditional "rosaries" such as the "Noah's ark rosary," the "goddess rosary," etc.

Program Overview:

To receive a complimentary ebook version of *The Rosary Workout,* send an email to contact@rosaryworkout.com with "Ebook Version" in the subject line. The ebook includes additional links and resources as well as color-coded graphics of the workouts. This offer is limited to those who have purchased this book or received it as a gift.

The Rosary Workout™ is divided into five parts. Parts I through IV relate important information on the Rosary and explain the principles of exercise science applied in the program. Part V contains the workouts. I know you are anxious to start the workout program, but it's very important that you read Parts I through IV first. Your success with The Rosary Workout™ begins with a thorough understanding of the Rosary and the 20 mysteries. Furthermore, you must understand a few concepts of exercise science in order to exercise safely and achieve maximum results.

Part I includes a brief but thorough study of the Rosary, its history, the significance of the Rosary prayers, and its power as an intercessory prayer.

Part II introduces the concept of the Rosary as Mary's School and the importance of Mary's role as advocate and teacher. You'll learn about the Nine Choirs of Angels and their significance in Rosary prayer.

Part III explains the scientific principles of exercise upon which I structured the workouts, along with information on nutrition and hydration.

Part IV will prepare you, physically and spiritually, to begin the workouts. This section adds suggestions on how to start and commit to The Rosary Workout™ and how to handle setbacks.

Part V contains the workouts. Graphics depicting the workout instructions are included for clarification.

The **Appendix** lists sources for obtaining a Rosary in various formats, a tutorial and graphic on "How to Pray the Rosary," a list of Rosary mysteries and the blessings and benefits of Rosary devotion, and exercise tips.

Program Definition and Goals:

There are nine levels of progression in The Rosary Workout™, each named after and dedicated to one of the Nine Choirs of Angels. The first three levels are designed for beginners, the middle three for intermediates, and the last three are advanced. Each level is four weeks long and presents a different set of goals for both physical and spiritual fitness.

The divisions of Beginner, Intermediate, and Advanced are based on both fitness ability and experience with meditation and Rosary prayer. That is, the Beginner Series is designed for someone who is a beginning exerciser and does not regularly pray the Rosary or has not practiced meditative prayer. The Intermediate and Advanced Series use the same method of placement in the program. Since few people fit neatly into one category in both areas, there are modifications throughout the program to accommodate those who fall under one level of physical fitness and another in Rosary prayer and meditation.

*Beginner Series...*A beginner is defined as a person who meets any of the criteria below:

- Has never exercised or has not exercised regularly in the last 6 months
- Is recovering from an injury
- Is pregnant or has given birth in the last 6 months
- Answered "Yes" to 2 or more PAR-Q questions on page 7
- Is under the age of 18 or over the age of 65
- Is under the care of a physician or psychiatrist/psychologist
- Does not regularly pray the Rosary
- Is not familiar with meditative prayer

Note: If you are a beginner to exercise, see your doctor before starting the program to determine any limitations or modifications.

Beginner Series Goals:

Angel Level: This is the most basic level, suited for anyone who is new to exercise and/or praying the Rosary. The goal is to memorize the Rosary prayers and to exercise while praying the Rosary twice a week.

Archangel Level: This is the beginning of integrating prayer, exercise and meditation. The goal is to practice Rosary meditation during exercise 2-3 days a week for 20-30 minutes. You'll also read passages from the Bible which describe the 20 mysteries of the Rosary.

Principality Level: This level introduces interval training as you continue practicing integrated exercise and meditation during 30-minute workouts, 3 days a week. You'll study artwork depicting the

Rosary mysteries as an aid to meditation.

Intermediate Series...An intermediate exerciser is defined as a person who meets the criteria below:

- Has completed the workouts of the Beginner Series **OR**
- Has exercised regularly (at least twice a week) for three months or more **AND**
      - Can exercise continually for 20 minutes or more
      - Prays the Rosary frequently or has memorized all the Rosary prayers
      - Is familiar with the 20 Rosary mysteries and their Biblical references
      - Has practiced meditative prayer
      - Is able to meditate during exercise

Intermediate Series Goals:

Power Level: This level is appropriate for an intermediate exerciser who is able to meditate on the Rosary mysteries during workouts. Weekly interval training is added, and workouts are planned 3 days a week for 30 minutes. Meditation is enhanced through an in-depth study of the Gospels that will continue through all three intermediate levels.

Virtue Level: This level builds on the Power Level workouts by increasing the intensity of interval training and adding a fourth day of exercise. An in-depth study of the Gospels continues.

Dominion Level: A new type of interval is added, and the workouts continue at 4 days a week for 30 minutes. The Gospel study is concluded.

Advanced Series...An advanced exerciser is defined as a person who meets the criteria below:

- Has completed the workouts of the Intermediate Series **OR**
- Is a competitive athlete in a sport that is conducive to the program
  (running, cycling, triathlon, swimming, etc.) **AND**
      - Has prayed the Rosary regularly
      - Is skilled at meditative prayer
      - Is able to meditate during exercise

Advanced Series Goals:

Throne Level: Exercise 4 days a week and increase interval duration and frequency. To improve spiritual fitness, I include recommendations for additional reading.

Cherubim Level: Workout frequency increases to 5 days per week and interval training intensifies. You'll reflect on the virtues or "fruits" of the Rosary mysteries and how to apply them in your daily life.

Seraphim Level: At this final level, you are ready to design your own workouts, incorporating exercise principles learned in The Rosary Workout™. You are encouraged to explore new ways to continue your study of the Rosary mysteries.

Part I:

The Rosary

Overview

History

Devotion

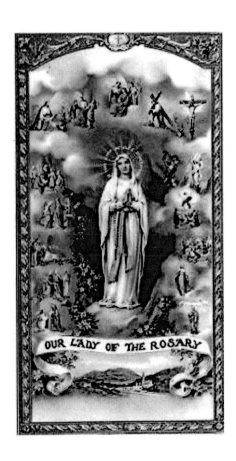

The Rosary, An Overview

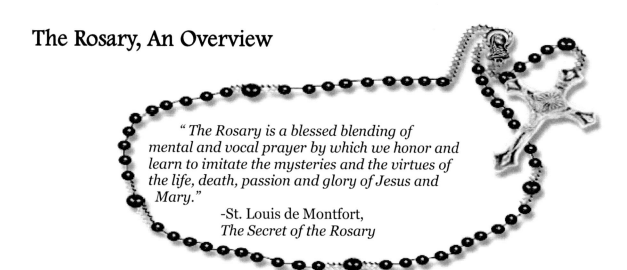

" The Rosary is a blessed blending of mental and vocal prayer by which we honor and learn to imitate the mysteries and the virtues of the life, death, passion and glory of Jesus and Mary."

-St. Louis de Montfort,
The Secret of the Rosary

The Rosary is both a mental and a vocal prayer. The vocal consists of saying the prayers (aloud or silently) that make up the Rosary: The Apostles' Creed, the Our Father, the Hail Mary, the Glory Be, the Hail Holy Queen and the Fatima Prayer. The vocal prayers are linked to the physical parts of the Rosary. The crucifix, beads, chains and central medal mark your "place" in the Rosary prayers. (See Appendix A-D for prayers and Rosary tutorial.)

The Rosary is not "vain repetition" as some would argue, but a means to concentrate our thoughts on the Gospels through Jesus' and Mary's examples of holiness. This reflection is the mental prayer, or meditation, and is the true "soul" of the Rosary. The decades of ten Hail Mary's serve as a type of background music to lull the mind into a meditative state. They mark the time allotted for meditation on each mystery, which represents a scene or event from the lives of Jesus and Mary.

A mystery was defined by the early Church as an event whose meaning can be partly understood on earth and partly understood in eternity. For instance, our human minds can understand the terror Jesus must have faced during the Agony in the Garden, yet we cannot fully comprehend how He took on the burden of all our sins. The mysteries of the Rosary are better understood through meditation and the Divine inspiration which can accompany it. Meditation during the Rosary is a skill which requires practice and focus, but is essential.

Each mystery also has an imbedded virtue, or "fruit" through which we can learn to imitate Christ. The Catechism defines virtue:

"A virtue is a habitual and firm disposition to do the good. It allows the person not only to perform good acts, but to give the best of himself. The virtuous person tends toward the good with all his sensory and spiritual powers; he pursues the good and chooses it in concrete actions. The goal of a virtuous person is to become like God." (CCC Section 1803)

Over time, a person who prays the Rosary devoutly and meditates on the 20 mysteries grows in and imitates these virtues.

A Rose Garden

The word "Rosary" comes from the Latin word rosarium, which means "a rose garden, often circular". In Catholicism, the images of a garden, a rose and a circle are rich in symbolism. To better understand this comparison, place a Rosary in front of you in a circle with the crucifix pointing toward you. The crucifix marks the opening prayer of the Rosary, The Apostles' Creed. The Creed (and our corresponding faith) is the key to unlock the garden gate, where Our Blessed Mother will lead us to a deeper understanding of the mysteries of the Rosary.

The five beads on the short chain, known as the pendant chain, represent stepping stones on a path leading into the garden. We pray an Our Father on the large bead, then three Hail Mary's on the smaller beads. These are traditionally prayed for an increase in the three theological virtues: Faith, Hope and Charity. The three beads are also said to honor the Three Persons of the Blessed Trinity: Father, Son and Holy Spirit.

We enter the garden, or circle of beads, when we begin the first decade of the Rosary. While we're in the garden, we meditate on five mysteries, leading us to a deeper understanding of the Gospels. We exit the garden after making a final prayer of praise and petition to our Blessed Mother, the Hail Holy Queen.

The Rosary is a path to the garden which we most long to enter: Paradise

Significance of the Rosary Prayers

The **Apostles' Creed** outlines the fundamental beliefs of Catholicism. It is an ancient prayer, dating back to the early Church and linked to Baptism. By reciting the Creed at the beginning of the Rosary, we renew the promises made at our own Baptism, affirm the truths of our faith, and set the proper tone for praying the Rosary.

It is most appropriate that the **Our Father** begins each decade of the Rosary. It is the prayer taught to us by Jesus Himself (Matthew 6: 9-13), and it focuses our attention to the heavenly origin of the mystery on which we are about to meditate.

The **Hail Mary** is the most recurrent prayer of the Rosary, prayed 53 times. Pope John Paul II emphasizes the link between the repeated Hail Mary's of the Rosary and their role in leading us to Jesus through Mary:

"The centre of gravity in the Hail Mary, the hinge as it were, which joins its two parts, is the name of Jesus. Sometimes, in hurried recitation, this centre of gravity can be overlooked, and with it the connection to the mystery of Christ being contemplated. Yet it is precisely the emphasis given to the name of Jesus and to His mystery that is the sign of a meaningful and

fruitful recitation of the Rosary." - Pope John Paul II, Apostolic Letter, *Rosary of the Virgin Mary*

The **Glory Be**, or Gloria, is a joyous praise and tribute to the Holy Trinity. It lifts our thoughts back to heaven after contemplating each mystery.

The **Fatima Prayer** is a fairly recent addition to the Rosary and was taught by the Blessed Mother herself to three children living in Fatima, Portugal. During a series of visions in 1917, Mary, calling herself the "Lady of the Rosary," encouraged daily recitation of the Rosary and asked that the following prayer be added to the end of each decade, following the Glory Be:

"Oh my Jesus, forgive us our sins. Save us from the fires of hell. Lead all souls to heaven, especially those in most need of thy mercy."

The central medal of the Rosary, usually portraying the Blessed Mother, is a marker for the **Hail Holy Queen** (an English translation of the Latin anthem, Salve Regina), a beautiful prayer of praise and petition to Our Lady, "*... the crowning moment of an inner journey which has brought the faithful into living contact with the mystery of Christ and His Blessed Mother.*" (Pope John Paul II, *Rosary of the Virgin Mary*)

Rosary Intentions: Increase the Power of Your Prayer

An intention is a favor or request. Just as you might pray an Our Father asking for the healing of a sick child, you can offer a Rosary for a certain intention. It may be as simple as praying for help in getting a promotion at work or as forthright as asking for world peace. Another common practice is to offer each decade of the Rosary for a different intention.

When you initially begin praying the Rosary, you will probably tend to focus your intentions on requests that affect you and your immediate family or friends, such as better health, more patience, a change of heart, etc. When you pray the Rosary more frequently, you can broaden your intentions to such causes as conversion of anonymous sinners who have no one to pray for them, an end to poverty, or other more global requests. The Rosary gives us the ability to bless others as well as ourselves!

The power of many people praying the Rosary for a single intention is staggering. Consider:

In 1571, at the Battle of Lepanto, a Christian naval force bravely fought the Turkish navy, who was trying to seize control of Europe. Outnumbered, the Christians had little hope of victory, but they did have a secret weapon — the Rosary. The sailors and devout Christians throughout Europe fervently prayed the Rosary throughout the battle. Miraculously, the Christians won a decisive victory, preventing Muslim control of Europe.

Centuries later, after World War II, control of Austria was given to Communist Russia. Ten percent of the people of this primarily Catholic country pledged to pray the Rosary in order to free their nation from Communist control. These Rosary crusaders persevered for over seven years until they were victorious. Russia abruptly and unexpectedly pulled out of Austria, baffling political analysts.

Rosary miracles abound even in our modern era. In 1964, the women of Brazil began a Rosary campaign to prevent a Communist takeover of their beloved nation. They organized Rosary marches and convinced millions to demonstrate peacefully through prayer, ultimately saving their country from Communism.

There are countless stories of miracles attributed to the Rosary, and those dedicated to the Rosary will often state that it has changed their lives. If you are interested in supporting a Rosary "crusade," a simple search online will yield many causes to join.

The History of the Rosary

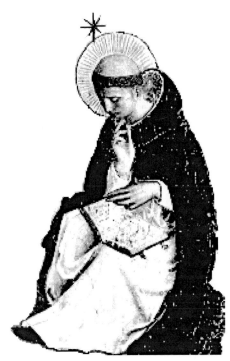

Saint Dominic

St. Dominic (1170-1221) is often known as the "Saint of the Rosary". In 1208, during a fervent prayer to combat the "Culture of Death" that existed during his time, he received a vision of our Blessed Mother, who said:

"Wonder not that you have obtained so little fruit by your labors-- you have spent them on barren soil, not yet watered with the dew of Divine Grace. When God willed to renew the face of the earth, He began by sending down on it the fertilizing rain of the Angelic Salutation. Therefore preach my Psalter [Rosary] composed of 150 Angelic Salutations and 15 Our Fathers, and you will obtain an abundant harvest."

Based on this revelation, St. Dominic spread devotion to the Rosary throughout Europe and eventually turned the tide against the "Culture of Death."

Although St. Dominic had a profound influence on the spread and devotion of the Rosary, its rich and complex history began before his time. The use of prayer beads is an ancient tradition practiced by many faiths. Prayer beads are used as a counting device and help establish a soothing rhythm of repeated prayer as an aid to meditation. In fact, the word "bead" comes from the Anglo-Saxon term "bede," meaning "prayer".

The Rosary, as we know it today, has evolved over centuries, but we can trace its roots to the Book of Psalms in the Old Testament. The Psalms, are considered to be a "School of Prayer" and contain songs of praise, lament and thanksgiving. Many are attributed to the ancestor of Jesus and Mary, King David.

The Psalms are filled with veiled prophecies on the life, death and Resurrection of Jesus and include many allusions to Mary. It was not until Jesus "opened the eyes" of His Apostles that these prophecies were understood:

"He said to them, 'These are my words that I spoke to you while I was still with you, that everything written about me in the law of Moses and in the prophets and psalms must be fulfilled.' Then he opened their minds to understand the scriptures." (Luke 24: 44-45)

Most Rosary historians first connect the Psalms to the Rosary in 9th century Ireland. During that time, Irish monks observed the common tradition in many monasteries of reciting the 150 Psalms from memory. The local lay people were inspired by this devout practice and wanted to emulate it, but they were unable to read or write. The monks suggested a simpler practice of reciting 150 Our Fathers, or Pater Nosters, to take the place of the Psalms. In order to keep track of the prayers, a string with 50 knots or pieces of wood was used. The 50 Pater Nosters were repeated three times, for a total of 150. This practice eventually spread throughout Europe. In fact, the strings of beads became known as "paternosters".

A devotion to Mary was gradually linked to the paternoster. Although the Hail Mary we pray today was not completed until the 15th century, it was a very common practice to recite the Angelic Salutation, or Ave, based on the words of the angel Gabriel to Mary in Luke 1:28 (with the later addition of the words of Elizabeth in Luke 1:42). Over time, 150 Angelic Salutations were prayed on the paternoster beads, and were known as "Our Lady's Psalter".

The 14th century brought another modification to the Rosary when a Carthusian monk, Henry Egher of Kalcar, divided the 150 Angelic Salutations into sets of 10 (called decades) with an Our Father between each decade. The Glory Be was added to the Rosary in the 15th century.

The 16th century essentially ended the evolution of the Rosary in its physical form. The pendant chain with five beads and a decorative ornament, along with a crucifix, was added. The Hail Mary, as we know it today, was complete and the tradition of praying the Apostles' Creed on the crucifix was commonplace. Finally, in 1573, the Council of Trent standardized the Rosary, calling it the "Dominican Rosary" in honor of St. Dominic. That same year, Pope Gregory XIII established the Feast of the Holy Rosary on the first Sunday of October. Since then, only minor changes have been made to the Rosary prayers, most regional or cultural.

The practice of meditating while praying the Rosary also evolved over centuries and, like the evolution of the Rosary beads, is rooted in the Psalms. During the Dark Ages, monks memorized and meditated deeply on the Psalms. They concentrated on the veiled, or hidden, prophecies written hundreds of years before Jesus fulfilled them in the Gospels. The monks wrote 150 Psalters, or praises, to honor Jesus based on their understanding of the Psalms. Over time, 150 additional Psalters were composed to honor Mary and served as tools for meditation while praying each the 150 Aves. This is one of the earliest links of meditation with Rosary prayer beads. An abbreviated version of 50 praises to Mary became known as a Rosarium, or bouquet or roses. Today, of course, it's called the Rosary.

The introduction of "Picture Rosaries" in the 15th century allowed the common people to practice meditating during repeated prayer. Since it was too expensive to print 150 pictures (one for each bead of the Rosary as used at that time), only 15 prints were made. These prints depicted various scenes of the gospels. People would gather to look at the pictures and meditate on each one in turn as they prayed one Our Father and ten Hail Mary's. St Louis de Montfort was especially devoted to this tool for meditation as it helped to focus the attention of his congregation.

The 15 scenes or events of the "Picture Rosaries" became known as the 15 mysteries of the Rosary and were standardized by Pope Pius V in 1569. Like the veiled prophecies of the Psalms, the mysteries of the Rosary are better understood through meditation and the Divine inspiration which accompanies it.

Our modern Rosary has been expanded to include a new set of mysteries, the Luminous Mysteries, instituted by Pope John Paul II in his apostolic letter on the Rosary. The five Luminous Mysteries complete the Rosary by adding events from Jesus' adult ministry. We now have 20 mysteries which focus our meditation on crucial events in the lives of Jesus and Mary.

Devotion to the Rosary

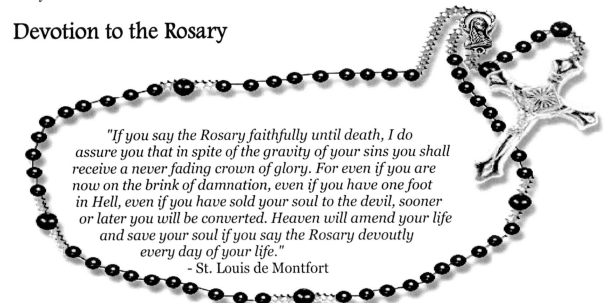

"If you say the Rosary faithfully until death, I do assure you that in spite of the gravity of your sins you shall receive a never fading crown of glory. For even if you are now on the brink of damnation, even if you have one foot in Hell, even if you have sold your soul to the devil, sooner or later you will be converted. Heaven will amend your life and save your soul if you say the Rosary devoutly every day of your life."
- St. Louis de Montfort

Countless saints, popes and lay people have been dedicated to the Rosary and its propagation throughout the world. Many miracles and life-changing events have been attributed to Rosary prayer and devotion.

I have already mentioned St. Dominic (1170-1221), "The Saint of the Rosary," and how he spread dedication to Mary's Psalter. He saw a vision of souls climbing to heaven, using the Rosary as a ladder. This vision was brought to life by Michelangelo in the Sistine Chapel through his masterpiece, "The Last Judgment," which shows two souls being lifted into heaven by a string of Rosary beads.

St. Dominic established an order of priests, the Dominicans, who are devoted to the Rosary and its proliferation, and are still active today. He also instituted the earliest form of a Rosary Confraternity (society devoted to a religious cause). It was called The Militia of Jesus Christ, and members recited The Psalter of Our Lady each day.

After St. Dominic's death, devotion to the Rosary slowly dwindled and nearly disappeared until the 15th century when a French Dominican priest, Blessed Alan de la Roche (also known as Alan de la Rupe), set the hearts of Christians on fire with a devotion to Our Blessed Mother and her most beloved prayer. He revived the Militia of Jesus Christ under the new title of Confraternity of the Most Holy Rosary. It still exists today, administered by the Dominican Order. Anyone willing to pray the 15 traditional mysteries of the Rosary each week may join, and will be abundantly blessed through this membership.
Visit their site: **www.rosary-center.org**

St. Louis de Montfort (1673-1716) was another champion of the Rosary. His book, *The Secret of the Rosary*, is essential reading for any student of this devotion.

Although these holy men lived long ago, devotion to the Rosary is still being spread in our time. St. Pio (1887-1968), known as Padre Pio, prayed multiple Rosaries daily and encouraged devotion to this Marian prayer. Most recently, Pope John Paul II (1920-2005), showed us how the Rosary is still very relevant through his many verbal and written testimonies. Our present pope, Benedict XVI, continues to emphasize the importance of the Rosary. These advocates place so much emphasis on praying the Rosary because there are abundant benefits and blessings available to those dedicated to this form of prayer.

Bishop Hugh Boyle (Bishop of Pittsburg) knew of the great power of devotion to the Rosary: *"No one can live continually in sin and continue to say the Rosary — either he will give up sin or he will give up the Rosary."*

It is possible to gain a plenary or partial indulgence by praying the Rosary. Although a discussion on indulgences is outside the scope of this book, you can learn more at these links:
www.ewtn.com/library/ANSWERS/INDULG.htm or
www.CatholicCulture.org (type "indulgence" in the Search box)

A complete list of benefits and blessings of Rosary devotion and Mary's promises to those devoted to the Rosary can be found in Appendix E.

Part II:

Mary's School

Our Advocate and Teacher

Angels and the Rosary

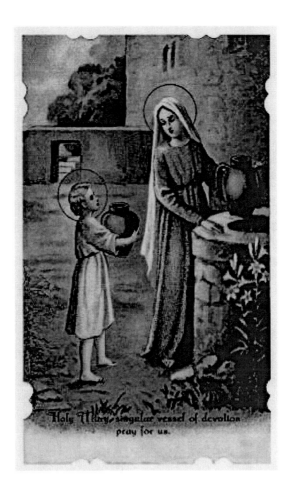

Holy Mary, singular vessel of devotion
pray for us.

Mary Is Our Advocate and Teacher

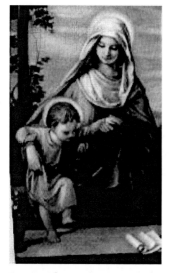

Mary's role as our advocate and teacher can be a confusing concept even to Catholics. Catholics do not worship Mary — that is reserved for the Three Persons of the Holy Trinity. We <u>honor</u> Mary as the greatest of saints due to her role as the Mother of our Savior.

Mary is our greatest advocate, presenting our prayers, requests and intercessions to her Beloved Son and pleading to Him on our behalf. We can find an example of the power of her assistance in the Gospel of John. "The Wedding Feast at Cana" relates Jesus' first miracle, turning water into wine. It's a familiar story to most Christians, but let's examine it more closely in the context of Mary acting as advocate. She presents a problem to her Son: The hosts, most likely friends of both Jesus and Mary, have run out of wine. This would be very embarrassing for them, and Mary knows that her Son can be of assistance. Jesus is reluctant to intervene, saying *"... My hour has not yet come."* (John 2:4) Yet Mary, demonstrating her great faith in Jesus' intervention, tells the servants, *"... Do whatever He tells you."* (John 2:5) Like the hosts of the wedding feast, we are able to tap into this marvelous wellspring of intervention through the Rosary. We present our petitions to the Blessed Mother, using her favorite prayer, and ask her to take them to her Son on our behalf.

Mary acts not only as advocate but also as our teacher:

"Christ is the supreme Teacher, the revealer and the one revealed. It is not just a question of learning what he taught, but of 'learning Him'. In this regard could we have any better teacher than Mary? ... Among creatures no one knows Christ better than Mary; no one can introduce us to a profound knowledge of His mystery better than His Mother." - Pope John Paul II, Apostolic Letter, *Rosary of the Virgin Mary*

Mary is the only human to be conceived without Original Sin, an event Catholics celebrate annually on December 8th, the Feast of the Immaculate Conception. No woman stained by sin would be worthy to give life to the Son of God. The Angel Gabriel greeted Mary with the words, *"Hail, full of grace..."* (Luke 1:28, Douay-Rheims edition). Sin takes away grace, yet Mary is *full* of grace, indicating that she is free from sin. Mary's state of grace is important because as Jesus' mother, she was also His primary teacher. Like any mother, Mary taught Jesus His first words, how to walk, and all the other basic skills a mother teaches a young child. She raised Him to adulthood and followed Him to the foot of the cross. She cherished every moment with her Son: *"... Mary kept all these things, reflecting on them in her heart."* (Luke 2:19)

Let's turn again to the story of "The Wedding Feast at Cana" to examine Mary's role as teacher. She *instructs* the servants at the wedding by stating, *"Do whatever He tells you..."*

These wise words still apply to us today. In the mysteries of the Rosary, Mary instructs and teaches us through the words and examples of her Son.

By praying the Rosary and meditating on the mysteries, we learn more about the life of Jesus through Mary's journey as our Savior's Blessed Mother. Mary, our teacher, leads us through the scenes of Jesus' conception, birth and childhood through the Joyful Mysteries. We follow along the path of His adult ministry through the Luminous Mysteries and witness the suffering of Jesus' Passion and Crucifixion as we contemplate the Sorrowful Mysteries. Finally, we rejoice in the glory of the risen Savior, the Holy Trinity and in Mary's role as Queen of Heaven and Earth through the Glorious Mysteries.

Those who study the mysteries through frequent and devout Rosary recitation are led to a search for deeper understanding of the Truth that Christ revealed and a desire to become more Christ-like. *"I will ponder your precepts and consider your paths."* (Psalm 119:15)

The School of Mary

With the Rosary, the Christian people sits at the school of Mary and is led to contemplate the beauty on the face of Christ and to experience the depths of His love. Through the Rosary the faithful receive abundant grace, as though from the very hands of the Mother of the Redeemer. - Pope John Paul II, Apostolic Letter, *Rosary of the Virgin Mary*

According to Robert Feeney, (author of The Rosary "The Little Summa") Mary's School of the Rosary has three levels: Beginner, Intermediate and Advanced. At the beginner stage, students learn the basic prayers of the Rosary, along with the mysteries. Meditation on the mysteries is a new skill that requires frequent practice to master.

The middle (or intermediate) class of Mary's school of the Rosary teaches students to attain a deeper knowledge by studying the Gospels. An intermediate student should not simply read the gospels, but truly study them by taking a Bible Study class, reading Catholic books on Bible interpretation or studying the works of the Early Church Fathers.

Finally, the highest (advanced) class of Mary's school leads the student to realize that the Rosary is a "rule of life" which challenges them to practice the virtues embedded in each mystery. These scholars are actually living the Gospels! Through many years of prayer and dedication to the Rosary, it is possible to model our own lives after those of Jesus and His Blessed Mother.

When you enroll in Mary's School of the Rosary, you are beginning an education that will last a lifetime. Imagine the rich blessings obtained through this school, whose graduates are granted "a never fading crown of glory" in heaven.

Angels and the Rosary

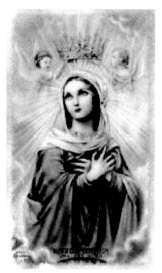

The presence of angels is invariably linked to the Rosary. Consider that the "Hail Mary" was previously known as the "Angelic Salutation" since it begins with the Angel Gabriel's words to Mary in Luke 1:28. One of Mary's many titles is "Queen of the Angels". As St. Louis de Montfort states in the *Treatise on the True Devotion to the Blessed Virgin*, "*Mary has authority over the angels and the blessed in heaven. According to St. Bonaventure, all the angels in heaven unceasingly call out to her: 'Holy, holy, holy Mary, Virgin Mother of God.' They greet her countless times each day with the angelic greeting, 'Hail, Mary', while prostrating themselves before her, begging her as a favor to honor them with one of her requests.*"

Pope Leo XIII elaborates the role of angels in the Rosary in his papal encyclical, *On the Confraternity of the Holy Rosary*:

"*... In reciting the Rosary, we meditate upon the mysteries of our Redemption... [and] in a manner emulate the sacred duties once committed to the Angelic hosts. The Angels revealed each of these mysteries in its due time; they played a great part in them; they were constantly present at them... What more divine, what more delightful, than to meditate and pray with the Angels? With what confidence may we not hope that those who on earth have united with the Angels in this ministry will one day enjoy their blessed company in Heaven?*"

Praying the Rosary devoutly can actually connect us with the holy angels. St. Alphonsus Liguori taught that by praying the Hail Mary, we attract the angels and repel the demons.

I chose to honor the role of angels in the Rosary by naming each of the nine levels of The Rosary Workout™ after one of the nine choirs.

The Nine Choirs of Angels

"Angel" is the Greek word for "messenger". This title refers to the office (or job) of angels, not their nature. The angels are spirits, created by God to serve Him. They watch over us and help guide us to heaven: "*For God commands the angels to guard you in all your ways.*" (Psalm 91:11) Angels are eager to help us and are powerful intercessors. We can pray for their assistance in the same way that we pray to Mary and the saints:

"*The smoke of the incense along with the prayers of the holy ones went up before God from the hand of the angel.*" (Revelation 8:4)

Some angelic scholars believe that the heavenly angels can be divided into nine choirs. There are Biblical references for each of these choirs, but most of our knowledge comes from St. Thomas Aquinas' work, *Summa Theologica*. He combined philosophy and Scripture to formulate conclusions on the nature, powers, and ranking of the angels.

Unlike the existence of angels in general, the division of the nine choirs is not an official Catholic doctrine. However, the concept does not contradict Church teachings and is mentioned in the writings of several Catholic saints. Angelic choirs are included in Catholic liturgy in the Preface of the Novus Ordo Mass:

"And so, with all the choirs of angels in heaven we proclaim your glory and join in their unending hymn of praise..."

<u>The Choir of Angels:</u>

Although the term "angel" is generally used to refer to all types of angels, there is a separate Choir of Angels. They are the lowest in the angel hierarchy, but are by no means unimportant. We are first introduced to the Choir of Angels in Genesis 16:7 when "God's messenger" appears to Hagar as she escapes the wrath of Abram's wife, Sarai.

The Angel Choir is part of the hierarchy of angels that is closest to the world of humans and material things. Scholars who study angels believe that most of our guardian angels come from this choir. They deliver messages from heaven and present our prayers to God.

<u>The Choir of Archangels:</u>

The archangels are probably the best-known type of angels. Archangel means "chief or leading angel". They may belong to this choir as well as other choirs. The only angels named in the Bible are archangels: Michael, Raphael and Gabriel. The book of Jude specifically describes Michael as an archangel (Jude 9), but Church tradition and liturgy assign this title to Raphael and Gabriel as well.

The term "archangel" is not introduced in the Bible until near the end of the New Testament: *"For the Lord Himself, with a word of command, with the voice of an archangel, and with the trumpet of God, will come down from heaven, and the dead in Christ will rise first."* (1 Thessalonians 4:16).

Like the Angel Choir, the Archangels are part of the hierarchy closest to the world of humans and material things. They guard humans who are tasked with important work in executing God's Divine Plan. They also watch over institutions of government and deliver the most urgent messages from heaven.

<u>The Choir of Principalities:</u>

The Principalities are the highest level in the hierarchy of the three angelic choirs closest to the world of humans and material things. Principalities are mentioned specifically by St. Paul: *"... The manifold wisdom of God might now be made known through the church to the principalities and authorities in the heavens."* (Ephesians 3:10)

The Principalities are tasked to guard and guide nations, kingdoms, states, cities, villages and towns. This choir is also believed to have been the source for many of the angels who followed Lucifer, or Satan, in rebelling against God: *"For our struggle is not with flesh and blood but with the principalities, with the powers, with the world rulers of this present darkness, with the evil spirits in the heavens."* (Ephesians 6:12) For this reason, we often refer to the angels who remained loyal to God as the "holy angels," as opposed to demons or devils.

The Choir of Powers:

The angelic Choir of Powers is the lowest in the middle hierarchy that is tasked with governing the cosmos. The Powers fight the forces of evil in the world. St. Paul mentions them, along with several other choirs, in his Letter to the Colossians: *"For in Him were created all things in heaven and on earth, the visible and the invisible, whether thrones or dominions or principalities or powers; all things were created through Him and for Him."* (Colossians 1:16)

In the same letter, St. Paul leads us to believe that like the Principalities, fallen angels also came from the Choir of Powers: *"[By] despoiling the principalities and the powers, [Christ] made a public spectacle of them, leading them away in triumph by it."* (Colossians 1:15)

The Choir of Virtues:

The second level of angels in the hierarchy that governs the cosmos is the Choir of Virtues. The Virtues control nature and the elements, and they aid in the working of miracles. St. Peter mentions this choir in his first letter:

"[Jesus Christ] is on the right hand of God, swallowing down death, that we might be made heirs of life everlasting: being gone into heaven, the angels and powers and virtues being made subject to him." (1 Peter 3:22, from the Douay-Rheims version of the Catholic Bible)

The Choir of Dominions:

The highest level of the middle hierarchy of the angels who govern the cosmos is the Dominion Choir (also known as Dominations). They are angels of leadership, wisdom, order and authority.

St. Paul teaches about Dominions in his Letter to the Ephesians: *"[Christ is seated] far above every principality, authority, power and dominion, and every name that is named not only in this age but also in the one to come."* (Ephesians 1:21)

The Choir of Thrones:

The uppermost hierarchy of angels are closest to God. They are called angels of pure contemplation. The lowest of these is the Choir of Thrones, angels of justice and humility.

"For in Him were created all things in heaven and on earth, the visible and the invisible, whether thrones or dominions or principalities or powers, all things were created through Him and for Him." (Colossians 1:16)

<u>The Choir of Cherubim:</u>

Cherubim are angels of intense knowledge of God. The word "cherubim" means "fullness of knowledge". They are the first angels mentioned in the Bible: *"When He expelled the man, He settled him east of the Garden of Eden; and He stationed the cherubim and the fiery revolving sword, to guard the way to the tree of life."* (Genesis 3:24)

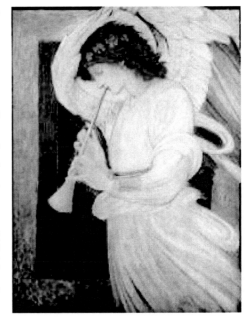

Golden cherubim adorned the Ark of the Covenant (Exodus 25:18-22) as well as the Temple of Solomon (1 Kings 6:23-28) and were vividly described in a vision to the prophet Ezekiel (Ezekiel 1:1-28).

<u>The Choir of Seraphim:</u>

Seraphim are the highest level of the Nine Choirs of Angels. They are closest to God and continually praise and glorify Him. "Seraphim" means "burning ones," and indeed they burn with love for God.

The prophet Isaiah was cleansed from sin by a Seraph (singular form of Seraphim) who touched a burning ember to his lips. Most Catholics will recognize the words of the Seraphim in Isaiah's vision from the Preface at Mass: *"'Holy, holy, holy is the Lord of hosts!' they cried one to the other, 'All the earth is filled with his glory.'"* (Isaiah 6:3)

Part III:

The School of *The Rosary Workout*™

Benefits of Regular Exercise

The Science of Exercise

Periodization

Exercise Fundamentals

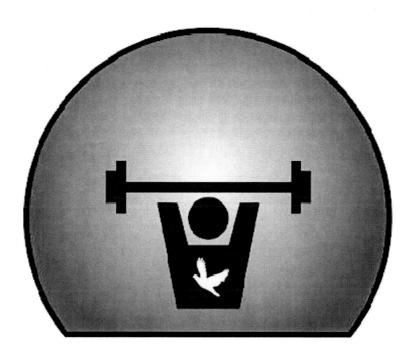

Benefits of Regular Exercise

Before I discuss the terminology, principles, and exercise science used to build The Rosary Workout™, I'd like to emphasize the physical benefits associated with any workout program.

There are countless scientifically-documented benefits to regular exercise! It's the closest thing we have to a "magic pill" and is available to anyone willing to make a commitment as low as 15-20 minutes just two to three days each week.

Exercise builds and maintains healthy muscles, bones, and joints. It decreases anxiety and depression and improves psychological well-being. Regular exercise enhances work, recreation, and sport performance and improves the quality of sleep. It reduces triglyceride levels (fat in the blood), increases HDL levels ("good" cholesterol) and aids insulin in removing excess sugar from the bloodstream

Exercise is powerful preventative medicine. It reduces the risks of and helps prevent heart disease, high blood pressure, high cholesterol, cancer, and type 2 diabetes to name a few.

People of all ages and walks of life benefit from exercise. It helps:
- Everyone to maintain a healthy body weight
- Older adults to become stronger, improve balance and mental function
- Pregnant women fight fatigue and stress and prepares them for delivery
- Women who've given birth return to their pre-pregnancy weight
- Men increase testosterone levels
- Children fight or prevent obesity

Regular exercise also:
- Prevents osteoporosis
- Controls the pain and joint swelling that accompanies arthritis
- Maintains lean muscle and bone mass, which is often lost with age
- Increases metabolism and regulates digestive functions
- Improves self-esteem and self-confidence
- Enhances clarity of thought and overall feelings of well-being and good health.

Exercise improves our quality of life and helps us live longer. It boosts energy and productivity so that we can accomplish more throughout the day. You are not being selfish or self-centered by setting aside a reasonable time for exercise! It is important to take care of the body created for you by God and to treat it with utmost respect, *"for we are fearfully and wonderfully made"*. (Psalm 139:14)

The Science of Exercise

There are four components to any exercise program: **frequency**, **intensity**, **duration** and **mode**. An effective program requires a systematic and logical manipulation of these components to produce a series of workouts that is varied, challenging and fun. The Rosary

Workout™ is designed to improve fitness using this approach.

Frequency: The number of training sessions or workouts in a given time period. The Rosary Workout™ begins at a frequency of just two days per week and gradually increases to five. I have included modifications throughout the program for those with limited time to exercise.

Intensity: The difficulty of the workout. This can be determined by heart rate, using a heart rate monitor, or by "perceived exertion". Perceived exertion assigns a subjective number to a level of intensity, using a scale of 1-10. A "1" on this scale is a state of rest (sitting in a chair reading a book) while a "10" marks an intensity that can be sustained for just a few seconds. The Rosary Workout™ uses the Perceived Exertion scale to determine intensity. I've included a short description of what each level of effort should "feel" like. The examples use walking/running, but the same idea can be applied to other forms of exercise.

Rating of Perceived Exertion Scale

1   **Very, Very Easy** (Sitting while reading or watching TV)

2   **Very Easy** (Strolling on a flat path or walking through a museum)

3   **Easy** (Walking a dog for exercise)

4   **Moderate** (Brisk walking)

5   **Somewhat Hard** (Jogging on a fairly flat or level surface)

6   **Hard** (Running on a fairly flat or level surface)

7   **Harder** (Running up a slight incline)

8   **Very Hard** (Briskly walking up stairs)

9   **Very, Very Hard** (Running up stairs)

10   **Maximal Effort** (Sprinting up stairs)

Beginners should strive for a rating of 2–4, while intermediate exercisers may boost their level of effort to a 5-7. Only advanced exercisers and competitive athletes should aim for the upper end of the scale, or 8-10.

Another method to evaluate exercise intensity is known as the "talk test". Most people pray the Rosary silently while exercising, or use a headset to listen to an audio Rosary, but you might occasionally say the prayers aloud to gauge intensity.

If you are able to exercise and recite an entire Rosary without effort, then you are probably exercising at a 3 or below on the RPE scale. On the other hand, if you can barely gasp out a few words, then your RPE is likely at 9 or above. The goal for moderate exercise is between the two extremes. You should be able to speak a few lines of the prayers without gasping for breath, which would correspond to a 4-6 on the RPE scale.

Intermediate and advanced exercisers can find the "talk test" helpful to gauge RPE during more strenuous workouts. If you're breathing fairly hard, but are still able to recite the prayers aloud, your RPE is probably in the range of 6 - 8. If you're gasping for air after every word, you're up to about an RPE of 9. If you can barely remember the prayers, let alone try to say them, you're at a 10.

Duration: The total time of the workout. Most experts agree that 10 minutes is really the minimum amount of exercise that can begin to be physiologically effective. Some studies have shown that 2 separate 10-minute sessions are just as effective as one 20-minute session. Beginners in The Rosary Workout™ start at a duration of 9 minutes. Advanced workouts can last as long as you have time to exercise. Most people can pray a Rosary in about 18-20 minutes, which makes it an ideal time marker for beginning exercisers.

Mode: The type of exercise chosen. Running, walking, jogging, swimming, hiking, biking, etc. are all different modes of rhythmic exercise which work well with The Rosary Workout™. Some modes of exercise are probably not suitable for the program. Team sports such as basketball, baseball, soccer, etc. provide too many distractions to meditative prayer. However, you can incorporate The Rosary Workout™ into your skill drills or conditioning exercises for team sports.

If you work out regularly, you probably have a pretty good idea of the mode of exercise you'll choose for The Rosary Workout™. But if exercise is a distant memory, or if you've started to exercise in the past and became bored or injured, you'll find some helpful suggestions in Appendix F.

Note: Unfortunately, non weight-bearing (non-impact) modes of exercise such as swimming, cycling, elliptical trainers, etc. do not increase bone density. If your primary mode of exercise is non weight-bearing, then it is important to add a day or two of strength training (weights, exercise tubes, body weight exercises such as push-ups, etc.) each week to avoid bone density loss. Another option is to cross-train by occasionally switching to a weight-bearing exercise such as walking or running.

Periodization

Periodization is a systematic approach to varying the volume and intensity of a training program in order to achieve optimum results. Many sports coaches and competitive athletes implement periodized workouts, but the concept can be applied to the recreational or beginning exerciser as well.

Periodization prevents random, unplanned and unstructured workouts as well as boredom, stagnation and plateaus. It eliminates a "stabbing in the dark" approach by providing a plan with goals and a means to achieve them. A lack of variety in exercise produces limited results. If you always walk the same distance at the same pace in the same amount of time, you'll reach a point where no improvements in fitness are made. Workouts that are always at an easy pace won't provide a challenge, yet a steady string of high-intensity workouts never allows for recovery and leads to burnout and possible injuries. Periodization solves these problems.

"Thus I do not run aimlessly! I do not fight as if I were shadowboxing. No, I drive my body and train it, for fear that, after having preached to others, I myself should be disqualified.
(1 Corintians 9:26-27)

The Rosary Workout™ uses a simple periodization model. Each of the nine levels is progressively more challenging, forming a **macrocycle** (or "large cycle"), lasting about nine months to a year. It's designed to bring a beginning exerciser to an advanced level. Progression through the entire macrocycle is not necessary. The program includes modifications to improve fitness without demanding more time for workouts.

The macrocycle consists of 3 **mesocycles** (or "medium cycles"), each lasting about three months. These are the Beginner, Intermediate and Advanced programs. Each has a defined structure and specific goals.

Finally, the mesocycles are subdivided into **microcycles** ("small cycles"), lasting 4 weeks. Intensity, frequency or duration increases slowly each week, with the third week as a "peak" week. The fourth week is relatively easy and is designed as a recovery. Each successive microcycle, or level, builds on the fitness gains made during the previous one.

Overload Principle *"For each shall bear his own load."* (Galatians 6:5)

In simple terms, the overload principle refers to making exercise harder by increasing the stress or load on the body during some type of work. For example, if you want to strengthen the bicep, or upper arm muscle, you might execute bicep curls with a 5-pound weight. When that becomes easy, the body has adapted and the muscle has grown stronger. To make the bicep even stronger, you would progress to using an 8-pound weight. You can continue to strengthen the bicep by increasing the weight used for the curls.

Since the heart is a muscle, an effective cardiovascular exercise program must make use of the overload principle in order to strengthen the heart and improve cardiovascular fitness. This applies not only to competitive athletes, but also to recreational exercisers, sedentary and disabled persons and even recovering cardiac patients. Obviously, you can't lift a dumbbell with your heart, so the overload principle is incorporated by making the heart work harder during exercise at an increased intensity. For example, if you normally walk during your workouts, you can overload the heart by "power walking," jogging, walking up a hill, etc.

The Rosary Workout™ incorporates the overload principle throughout the program using the periodization model outlined above. Once again, structure is important. You don't want to do an "overload" workout every day, nor do you want to limit them to once in a blue moon. A systematic approach is needed — there has to be a plan. Recovery is also important (see discussion below). If overload is not followed by recovery, then the body will never get adequate rest to grow stronger. Adaptation occurs during recovery, not during the overload. Adaptation means that the body gets "used" to the exercise, so it becomes easier. After adequate recovery and adaptation, the body is once again ready for another overload workout. Using this approach systematically and carefully results in a continual improvement in fitness.

Recovery: *"... He rested on the seventh day from all the work He had undertaken."* (Genesis 2:2)

The Rosary Workout™ uses the term "recovery" in three ways. First, it refers to a rest period after an overload. "Rest" in this application is not stopping and sitting on a park bench, but rather a slowdown of the pace or intensity. This allows you to catch your breath and takes the stress off the heart muscle. The period of recovery is usually longer than the amount of time spent in overload, but it can be varied based on training goals.

Secondly, "recovery" refers to a low-intensity workout done the day after an overload workout. Studies have shown that this "active recovery" or "active rest" workout is better than taking a day off from exercise. The theory is that by increasing blood circulation through a low-intensity workout, the body is better able to remove the exercise by-products that cause the "burn" or soreness in the muscles. Muscle soreness can be further reduced by stretching after the recovery workout.

Finally, the term "recovery" refers to a relatively easy week of workouts following a challenging or "peak" week of workouts, using the periodization model.

The application of recovery is essential in preventing injury, illness and overtraining.

Interval training:

Interval training is an application of the overload principle. An interval is a short bout of increased intensity, followed by a period of recovery, or rest. Interval training can be random ("Race you to the next sign!") or very structured. Typically, the interval is short and the recovery somewhat longer.

The Rosary Workout™ uses structured intervals and recoveries, based on the prayers of the Rosary. This approach enables the exerciser to experience the benefits of interval training without interrupting the prayerful meditation of the Rosary.

Many studies show that interval training is a very effective method to improve cardiovascular fitness. There are several advantages to this type of workout.

Intervals:

- Are ideal for workouts where one is pressed for time
- Increase the number of calories burned
- Improve speed and overall fitness
- Can be used by competitive athletes and recreational exerciser
- Utilize a combination of two of the body's fuel sources: stored fat and glycogen
  (carbohydrates stored in the muscles and liver)

Although beneficial, interval workouts should not be overdone or they can lead to injury or overtraining. The periodization approach used in The Rosary Workout™ ensures that the exerciser is well-prepared for intervals when they're introduced and that adequate recovery occurs before another session of interval training.

Overtraining:

Overtraining is the result of too much exercise with inadequate recovery. You're essentially pushing yourself too hard. Although The Rosary Workout™ is designed to avoid overtraining, sometimes added stresses such as psychological stress at home or work, exercising in extreme heat or cold, poor diet or sleep habits, illness, etc. can contribute to overtraining.

There are several symptoms that may indicate overtraining:

- Feeling of sluggishness or lethargy
- Restless sleep or insomnia
- Loss of appetite
- Frequent colds or illness
- Elevated heart rate upon waking
- Decreased performance during workouts or lack of motivation to exercise
- Irritability
- Muscle soreness that won't go away or minor injury that won't heal

The cure for overtraining is to take about three to five days off from all exercise. Get extra sleep by going to bed early, sleeping in or napping. Eat a healthy diet and try to minimize stress. If you are injured, visit a physician and ask for specific instructions for exercise modifications or request a referral to a physical therapist.

To prevent overtraining, do not deviate excessively from the workout plan. Keep a detailed journal and review it frequently. You'll be able to see the initial symptoms of overtraining so that you can back off a bit. Furthermore, you'll discover what stresses your body can handle and develop an awareness of when you're doing too much.

Exercise Fundamentals

The warm-up, cool-down and a post-exercise stretching session are fundamental parts of the overall workout. The warm-up prepares the body physiologically and psychologically for exercise and reduces the risk of injury. The cool-down at the conclusion of the workout is essential to prevent blood from pooling in the lower part of the body and causing dizziness or even fainting. A post-exercise stretching session improves range of motion, reduces muscle soreness and aids in relaxation.

Warm-Up:

It is very important to begin every workout with an adequate warm-up to prevent injury and prepare the body for more vigorous exercise. A warm-up also prepares the mind for the challenge of more strenuous exercise. By beginning a workout with a few minutes of low-intensity exercise, you literally warm your body by increasing the core temperature. The warm-up exercise should involve the same major muscles used during the main workout. For example, if you will be running, warm up with a brisk walk or an easy jog.

A warm-up will:

- Increase blood flow to the working muscles, improving their elasticity
- Increase the body's core temperature, allowing muscles to contract more forcefully and relax quickly
- Increase metabolic rate
- Shut off blood flow to the stomach, preventing nausea and indigestion
- Increase range of motion
- Prepare the body for more intense exercise
- Prevent injury through a gradual increase in intensity
- Dilate blood vessels to reduce stress on the heart

Ideally, a warm-up should last about 5-10 minutes for a workout of 30 minutes or longer. Shorter workouts still require a warm-up, but it can be decreased to 3-5 minutes if the main workout is fairly low-intensity.

Research shows that stretching after a warm-up is not really beneficial, and in fact practically negates all the benefits of the warm-up since your body returns to its resting state as you stretch. The best time to stretch is at the end of a workout when your muscles are warm and pliable.

Since The Rosary Workout™ is an integrated approach to care of the soul and the body, I will also stress the importance of a spiritual "warm-up". As you prepare the body for exercise, you should simultaneously prepare the mind for prayer. During your physical warm-up, take a few minutes to think about your Rosary intentions as well as the Rosary mysteries upon which you will meditate. It is helpful to ask your guardian angel, a patron/favorite saint, the Blessed Mother or the Holy Spirit to help you focus on prayer and meditation during your workout.

Base Pace:

I use a term called "base pace" to describe an intensity, or RPE, that can be maintained for the duration of a given workout. This pace should be "comfortably uncomfortable". That is, it should not be so easy that it can be maintained for over an hour, but it does make you work a bit.

There is a point during exercise at which you reach your "lactate threshold" or LT. (It's also commonly called "anaerobic threshold".) This is the point where your body can no longer process exercise by-products, and they begin to accumulate in the bloodstream. You begin to feel a "burn". Exercise scientists are still trying to determine exactly what causes this burn, but LT is used as a marker for this transition.

Base pace is an exercise intensity below lactate threshold. If you start feeling the "burn" in your muscles, then slow your pace a bit. Another simple test is to close your mouth and breathe through your nose. If you are forced to open your mouth to get air, then you're likely exercising above lactate threshold.

Cool-down:

A cool-down at the end of a workout is just as important as a warm-up. An effective cool-down has four components: low-intensity exercise, stretching, hydration and refueling. The first two components are discussed below. Nutrition and hydration are covered in the next section.

Following the main workout, reduce the exercise intensity so that your heart rate and rate of breathing slow down gradually. This prevents blood from pooling in the legs which can lead to dizziness or fainting. It also aids the body in processing the exercise by-products, which cause the "burning" sensation in tired muscles. Furthermore, the decreased pace and intensity signal the body to return blood flow to the stomach and intestines to aid in digestion and a return of appetite. The cool-down period should last at least 3-5 minutes. Extend the time to 5-10 minutes or more after longer or very high-intensity exercise.

During the physical cool-down period, finish your prayer and meditation or just enjoy your surroundings and the great feeling of having completed a spiritual workout.

Stretching:

Stretching helps to reduce muscle soreness and prevent injury. The ideal time to stretch is immediately after the cool-down period. The muscles are warm and pliable and less likely to be injured. Stretch all the major muscles used during the workout. You should feel a gentle pull in the muscle, never a sharp pain. Don't bounce or hold your breath, and hold each stretch for at least ten seconds. Holding a stretch for a longer period (45 seconds or more) allows you to gently deepen the stretch, improving flexibility and range of motion.

If you don't have time to stretch immediately after your workout, try to make time later in the day. Before stretching, warm up with a few minutes of low-intensity exercise as you should never try to stretch a "cold" muscle. Recent studies have shown that it doesn't matter so much <u>when</u> you stretch but rather <u>that</u> you stretch, preferably 20-30 minutes weekly.

I recommend the book, *Stretching* by Bob Anderson, as an excellent resource. Most libraries carry a copy.

Nutrition and Hydration for Exercise

Your body's "engine" needs a bit of fuel, in the form of food, to get you through a workout. It's important to eat before and after exercise. Ideally, you should eat a small meal/snack of whole-grain carbohydrates and quality protein about 1-2 hours before your workout. Of course, if you are planning to exercise before work at 5:30 am, this is not realistic. In this case, eat a very light carbohydrate snack such as half a piece of wheat toast, a mini bagel, 1-2 mini waffles, a fig bar, granola bar, etc. Early-morning exercisers should increase the warm-up time to ensure that blood flow to the stomach is cut off to prevent stomach cramps or a feeling of nausea.

It is also important to "refuel" post-workout. A light snack or meal that includes whole-grain carbohydrates and a quality protein eaten within 45 minutes after exercise will optimize replacement of glycogen stored in the muscles. Below are a few suggestions for healthy pre- and post-workout snacks:

- Old-fashioned oatmeal with walnuts and blueberries
- Whole-grain waffle spread with natural peanut butter and a little syrup
- Whole-grain cereal with low-fat milk
- One or two scrambled eggs in a small tortilla with salsa
- Whole grain mini pancakes
- ½ English muffin with real fruit spread or natural peanut butter
- Low-fat cottage cheese with fruit
- Apple slices spread with natural peanut butter or soft cheese
- Grapes and a slice of cheese
- Fresh fruit and a handful of walnuts or almonds
- Celery sticks spread with natural peanut butter or low-fat cream cheese
- Vegetables with low-fat dip or hummus
- Tuna and low-fat mayonnaise on whole-grain crackers
- ½ a deli sandwich with low-calorie spread on whole-grain bread
- Granola bar and an orange or tangerine

Diets:

It's not a great idea to start a new diet at the same time you start a new exercise program. Studies have concluded that this is just too much restriction to work for the long term. I recommend changing one thing at a time. Wait until you have already established a regular exercise habit before you make major changes to your diet. Even then, you should consult your physician first. Of course, if you decide to pass on the donuts after Mass because you've been working so hard on your fitness goals, then feel free! In fact, studies show that people who start, and stick to, an exercise program actually change their eating habits to reflect healthier choices.

Hydration:

Proper hydration is essential to enjoyable and effective workouts. Water is the best fluid for shorter workouts. Try to drink at least 8-16 oz. of water within an hour of the start of your workout. If you are exercising longer than 15 minutes or if you'll be outside in hot or humid weather, take along a water bottle and sip from it throughout your workout. For workouts longer than 45 minutes or very intense shorter workouts, many experts advise using a diluted sports drink. Hydration should continue after your workout. It's helpful to keep a glass or bottle of cold water nearby throughout the day so you can continually sip from it.

Part IV:

Prerequisites

Proper Time and Season

Discipline

Setbacks and Solutions

Keeping Track of the Rosary Prayers While Exercising

Role Models

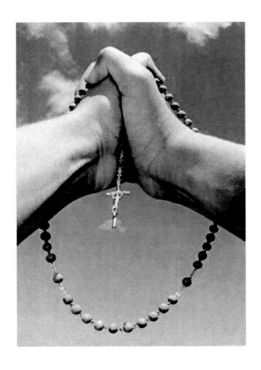

Proper Time and Season

"There is an appointed time for everything, and a time for every affair under the heavens." (Ecclesiastes 3:1)

Before you begin The Rosary Workout™, I encourage you to evaluate your present level of exercise and the demands on your time. If you are currently exercising regularly (at least twice a week for a minimum of 20 minutes), then it will be a fairly simple matter to start The Rosary Workout™ program.

However, if you are a beginning exerciser (or if exercise is a distant memory), then take a good, hard look at your lifestyle. Be realistic; don't set yourself up for failure. If there is a deadline looming, or a major event or holiday, you may want to wait until the event has passed. Get out your calendar or planner and schedule a date to begin the program.

If you can't find 10-20 minutes twice a week to exercise, then ask yourself what is making you so busy that you neglect your own health and spiritual needs? Pray for the courage and commitment to begin the program. You CAN do this! When you are ready to start the program, resolve to make a commitment to at least get through the 12-week Beginner level.

The Beginner Level of The Rosary Workout™ requires a minimal time commitment. The primary objective of this level is to make exercise a habit and an essential part of your lifestyle that you look forward to and enjoy.

Examinations of the Body and Soul

Another important step to complete before beginning the program is to evaluate both your physical and spiritual health. Care of the body and care of the soul go hand in hand, and an examination is a good starting point.

To evaluate your physical health, make an appointment with your physician. He or she will perform an examination and review your medical history to determine your readiness for exercise, as well as any limitations. Bring a list of recent or past injuries, illnesses, etc. and any exercise-related questions. If you are on medications, ask your doctor if they will have an impact on your exercise program. Certain medications affect heart rate, so in this case, it is important to rely on the Rating of Perceived Exertion (RPE) scale mentioned earlier in the book rather than a heart rate monitor.

To evaluate your spiritual health, you should visit a priest in the sacrament of Confession or Reconciliation. Before you do this, you must first examine your conscience. You may not have heard this term since second grade, but a thorough examination of conscience is a crucial part of the sacrament of Reconciliation.

If you are at a loss as to how to do this, there are many good books and pamphlets on the subject. Check your local Catholic bookstore, parish gift shop, the pamphlet rack in the back of some Catholic churches, or the internet.

I know this is a big and difficult step for many people — both going to the doctor and going to Confession -- but it is an important one. You will receive so many more benefits from The Rosary Workout™ with a clean bill of health and a "clean" soul.

Discipline

"Every athlete exercises discipline in every way. They do it to win a perishable crown, but we an imperishable one." (1 Corinthians 9:25)

In order to become a model student and to graduate from any type of school, a certain level of discipline is required. Those devoted to the Rosary know that it takes discipline to focus on the mysteries and to avoid distraction. Similarly, those committed to lifelong fitness have the discipline to exercise when they'd rather sit in front of the TV. The Rosary Workout™ program does require discipline. Although the time commitment is initially low (about 10-20 minutes, twice a week), you will need to discipline not only your body but your mind as well. It takes concentration and focus to pray and exercise at the same time, but the benefits are well worth it.

Discipline in Exercise Adherence:

Fitness professionals refer to exercise adherence as a person's ability to execute an exercise program, or "stick-to-it-iveness". This is one of the biggest obstacles facing beginners. There are four primary factors that affect exercise adherence: injury, time, boredom and results. The Beginner Level of The Rosary Workout™ is designed with these factors in mind to assist beginners in developing a habit of regular exercise. Here are a few tips to help with exercise adherence:

1. **Keep an exercise journal.** This can be anything from an elaborate computer program to a simple spiral notebook. You will use this journal to list your goals, give a brief description of your workout and how you felt, and any other pertinent notes. Studies show those who keep records have the greatest success in sticking to an exercise program.

2. **Schedule your workouts as if they were appointments**. Find time in your week and write a note on your calendar or planner. It's a good idea to schedule an alternate day so you have a fallback.

3. **Exercise in the morning if possible**. Studies show that morning exercisers have the greatest rate of success, but exercise at any time of day will work if you have a plan and stick to it.

4. **Ask for the support of your family**. Let your family members know that you have made a commitment to exercise and tell them that you need their help and encouragement. Explain that your improved health will give you more energy to meet their needs. If possible, recruit your family to join you in The Rosary Workout™ program.

5. **Pray for help**. Most secular exercise books and fitness programs omit this powerful tool

for exercise adherence. Your body is God's masterpiece, and He expects you to take care of it. Pray to Jesus, the Blessed Mother, St. Sebastian (patron saint of athletes), your personal patron saint, your guardian angel — the list is endless — for help. Ask others to pray for your success: *"The fervent prayer of a righteous person is very powerful."* (James 5:16)

6. **Find a workout partner**. It's much easier to follow through with your workout plan if you know that another person will be waiting for you. A workout partner enables you to pray the Rosary together, taking turns leading the prayers. You'll have the added benefit of Jesus' presence: *"For where two or three are gathered together in my name, there am I in the midst of them."* (Matthew 8:17) Ask a family member or friend to be your workout partner, or put a notice in your parish bulletin. If you can't find a workout partner, a commitment to walk the family dog or a friend's dog twice a week might get you out the door. You certainly don't need a workout partner every time you exercise, but it helps to have another person's encouragement and motivation.

7. **Keep a gym bag or walking/running shoes in your vehicle at all times**. You never know when you might get a chance to exercise. If a meeting or appointment is canceled, get out your walking or running shoes and use the time to get some exercise. Park 5-10 minutes from your destination and walk — this is a great way to exercise before and after daily Mass if you are able to attend.

8. **Try a little redemptive suffering**. There will be days when it's too hot or it's raining outside or perhaps you're tired and just plain don't feel like exercising. In this situation, follow the example of the saint known as "The Little Flower," St. Therese of Lisieux, and practice a little redemptive suffering. Redemptive suffering means to "offer up" physical or mental suffering or even little annoyances to God. St. Therese wrote of the "little ways" she turned life's minor difficulties into acts of love for God. You can "offer up" your discomfort for the redemption of your own soul or for a prayer intention for another person. Of course, if you experience genuine pain while exercising, you should stop immediately and see a doctor or call 911 if needed. Similarly, if you're experiencing overtraining symptoms, then rest is the best antidote. I'm not advocating a "no pain, no gain" approach. Instead, I encourage you to "offer up" the inconvenience of exercising when you don't feel like it.

9. **Reward success**. Rewards usually follow discipline and commitment. An important motivator is to set a reward for your hard work. Before you begin each level of The Rosary Workout™, determine an appropriate reward to aid you in reaching your goals. Ideas for rewards include:

- New workout shoes or apparel
- A new Rosary CD or Bible
- Gym membership or a few sessions with a personal trainer
- A medal with an image of Mary, Jesus, or your patron saint
- A massage, manicure or pedicure
- A long soak in the tub or an afternoon nap
- A new book or simply a gold star in your journal

Discipline in Praying and Meditating on the Rosary:

The Catholic Catechism states that *"Meditation is above all a quest. The mind seeks to understand the why and how of the Christian life, in order to adhere and respond to what the Lord is asking. The required attentiveness is difficult to attain [but] we are usually helped by books ...especially Sacred Scripture."* (CCC Section 2705)

Meditation on the mysteries of the Rosary differs from the New Age notion of meditation or "centering prayer". The mysteries of the Rosary direct our focus to Christ while New Age meditation focuses on self.

St. Louis de Montfort makes this clear by stating the results of prayerful Rosary meditation in *The Secret of the Rosary*:

- It gradually gives us a perfect knowledge of Jesus Christ
- It purifies our souls, washing away sin
- It gives us victory over our enemies
- It makes it easy for us to practice virtue
- It sets us on fire with love of Jesus
- It enriches us with graces and merits

Meditation, like any skill, requires practice and study. It's not a linear progression, but a journey. At first, you will probably experience difficulty focusing on the Rosary mysteries. You may not understand what meditation is and why the mysteries have any impact on your life in the modern world.

The spiritual exercises in the Rosary Workout™ are designed to help you on your journey in meditative prayer. The Beginner Series focuses on the basics: learning the Rosary prayers, reading the Bible references for each mystery, and studying artwork that depicts the mysteries. This provides a starting point for meditation and helps form a mental picture of each mystery.

By imagining yourself as an observer of the event, you can watch the scene unfold like a movie. It may be a very short movie, but it's definitely a beginning. I occasionally incorporate my exercise into the scene. For example, I'll imagine that I'm hiking behind Mary as she journeys to the hill country to visit Elizabeth in The Visitation. I try to focus on Mary's humility and charity in hurrying to help her cousin cope with a pregnancy in old age.

The next step on your journey to meaningful Rosary meditation is to expand the mental picture by placing the events of the mysteries in the context of Salvation History — the story of God's Divine Plan to save humanity from the consequences of sin. Obviously, the primary source for such a study is the Bible. Therefore, the spiritual exercises of the Intermediate Series require an in-depth study of the four Gospels. Although simply reading the Gospels is a good start, you will understand so much more through a guided study. Expanding your Bible study to include the rest of the Bible will only add to your comprehension. For example, you'll learn that the First Joyful Mystery, The Annunciation, is rooted at the beginning of the Bible, in the third chapter of Genesis. In fact, all the Rosary mysteries have roots in the Old Testament. By studying Salvation History, you'll discover how Jesus and the events of the Gospels are a fulfillment of the Old Testament.

Bible study will help you advance in Mary's School of the Rosary. Meditative prayer becomes easier when you include more than just a mental picture of the Rosary mysteries. You may find that your study efforts are rewarded with Divine Inspiration. These gifts of grace occur when you experience a sudden revelation that helps you to better understand the mystery you're pondering. It's an exhilarating feeling, and it fuels your eagerness to keep studying, reading and learning.

I was once meditating on The Birth of Jesus, when I began to think of the birth of my own children. I recalled the joy of meeting each child in the delivery room and my ever-increasing love as they grew. I was suddenly struck with an awareness of the depth of love that Mary and Jesus must have for each other. Since they were both free from Original Sin, there were no obstacles of selfishness, laziness, resentment or other human weakness to impede their love. This must have been God's vision of love between mother and child when he created Adam and Eve. I began to experience a deeper appreciation for the great bond between Jesus and His beloved mother.

Unfortunately, not every session of meditative prayer is blessed with such gifts of grace. There will be plenty of instances when you realize that you've been "meditating" on your plan for dinner tonight or a problem at work. You may find that certain mysteries just don't make sense to you. This is part of the journey. Pray for help, and it will come. I struggled with one particular mystery for quite some time. I even thought about it when I wasn't praying the Rosary. I finally prayed for help. The next week, just one sentence in the priest's homily at Mass unlocked the mystery for me to the extent that I look at the world with an entirely different view.

The more you study and meditate, the more you'll realize that the Rosary mysteries are an infinitely deep well from which you can draw a never-ending supply of knowledge. Expand your study by reading commentaries on the Rosary such as those by St. Louis de Montfort, Pope John Paul II, Robert Feeney, Scott Hahn, and many others. As you read and research, you'll build a wealth of knowledge and understanding to reflect upon as you pray the Rosary.

The final step is to put your meditative prayer into practice. At this point, you're actually learning to live the Gospels by following the examples of virtue portrayed in the Rosary mysteries. The Rosary becomes a "rule of life" that governs all your thoughts, words and actions.

The Advanced Series provides assignments to continue your progress in Mary's School, but few people are able to truly live the message of the Gospels every day. Even the Apostles and the great saints faltered now and then. Don't let this discourage you! Everyone can experience "moments of greatness" in which they become Christ-like in thought, word and deed.

A few more ideas:

It may be helpful to compile a personal Rosary notebook. This is an effective tool to aid your progress through Mary's School of the Rosary. A simple beginning is to divide your notebook into the Joyful, Sorrowful, Glorious and Luminous Mysteries. Add inspiring passages from Scripture based on your own reading or by searching through the countless Rosary books, pamphlets and websites which include Biblical quotations. You might include beautiful or inspiring artwork depicting the mysteries. Record the details of any revelations you received. As you grow spiritually, expand your notebook as needed.

If you are new to spiritual meditation, read through the helpful articles in the *Catechism of the Catholic Church* Part Four: Christian Prayer. If you don't own a copy of the *Catechism*, search the internet for an online version.

I have listed various books, pamphlets and websites throughout this book that I have personally found helpful in my study of the Rosary. Check the Appendix for more resources.

Setbacks and Solutions

"Look to yourselves that you do not lose what we worked for but may receive a full recompense." (2 John 1:7)

It happens to all of us eventually: We begin a program for positive change, things go well for a time, and then we slide back into our old habits. This can be very discouraging, but it's important to view such slip-ups as a challenge. Consider that forming a new habit can take weeks or even months. Setbacks are a natural part of this process.

Since The Rosary Workout™ includes both physical and spiritual challenges, I'll address the common causes of setbacks to the care of the body and of the soul. I offer solutions to help get you back on track.

Setbacks in Care for the Body: Lapses and Relapses:

New exercise programs are especially prone to setbacks known as lapses and relapses. A lapse is a single slip-up such as skipping a workout and not re-scheduling it later in the week. A lapse is certainly not a problem, as long as you return to your workouts. A day or even a week off now and then is very beneficial in an exercise program. The Rosary Workout™ has built-in breaks and options to work out fewer days than planned in order to prevent lapses. A lapse becomes a problem when it turns into a relapse, or a return to the "old" behavior (not exercising at all or very sporadically).

To prevent a relapse, formulate a plan for events or seasons that you know will be stressful. For instance, many people stop exercising from Thanksgiving to Christmas. They claim they will begin in January, but something else comes up and the day to start exercising again is put off indefinitely.

Since The Rosary Workout™ includes planned workouts for 36 weeks, it is possible to compare the workout plans to your calendar or schedule. If you know that a difficult time is coming up (Thanksgiving, summer vacation, family visit, etc.) then simply cut back the workouts to a number that is feasible. It's also possible to shorten the workouts. It only takes about 18-20 minutes to pray a Rosary during exercise, and a short Rosary Workout break during a stressful day can help clear your head.

An exercise journal is another great tool to help work through a relapse. Review your journal for clues as to why you stopped exercising. Were the workouts too hard or too easy? Was soreness, injury or illness a factor? Did you stop scheduling your exercise sessions in the hope of trying to fit them in? Look for positive notes in your journal to rediscover the benefits of regular exercise.

The preceding section on Discipline lists additional suggestions for exercise adherence to prevent lapses and relapses. Don't forget the power of prayer to assist you in returning to your good habits!

Setbacks in Care for the Soul: Spiritual Dryness *"At once the Spirit drove Him out into the desert."* (Mark 1:12)

When you start praying the Rosary regularly, you may find that blessings seem to literally rain down upon you. You feel genuinely happy and begin to search out other ways to enrich your spiritual life. Perhaps you start going to daily Mass or reading about the lives of the saints. You begin to truly feel the presence of the Lord and His Blessed Mother. There's a sense of peace, excitement and joy. Then suddenly, almost abruptly -- nothing. Your prayers seem pointless, you're easily distracted and you may even begin to wonder if there really IS a God.

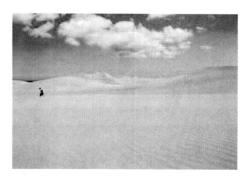

The *Catechism* addresses this topic: *"[A] difficulty, especially for those who want to pray, is dryness... when the heart is separated from God, with no taste for thoughts, memories, and feelings, even spiritual ones."* (*CCC* Section 2731)

Many people experience this spiritual dryness or the "dark night of the soul" where God's presence is no longer felt. Even the great saints endured this trial. Recently, it was discovered that a holy woman in our modern era, Blessed Teresa of Calcutta (often known as "Mother Teresa"), spent most of her life in the "dark night of the soul," yet she continued her dedication to prayer and helping the poorest of the poor. Think of dryness as time spent in the desert just as Jesus Himself did.

It's important that you continue to pray. Seek the advice of a trusted priest or bring up your difficulties during Confession. You may find it helpful to read about saints who wrote about this topic, such as St. John of the Cross and St. Teresa of Avila.

This period of dryness won't last forever. God has not forgotten you. If you persevere in faith and humility, you'll receive the refreshing rain of grace that comes after time spent in a spiritual desert.

In the meantime, follow the advice of "The Little Flower," St. Therese of Lisieux: *"When I am in this state of spiritual dryness, unable to pray or to practice virtue, I look for little opportunities for the smallest trifles to please Jesus, such as a smile, a kindly word when I would rather be silent... If no such occasion offers itself, I try at least to say over and over again that I love Him."* Letter from St. Therese to her sister, Celine, August 2, 1893

Keeping Track of the Rosary Prayers While Exercising

I have prayed the Rosary while exercising for many years and have tried various means of keeping track of the prayers. One solution is to carry a 5-decade Rosary. A modern-day example can be found in Blessed Pier Giorgio Frassati, a young Italian athlete who lived in the early 1900's. He often walked the streets of his village, Rosary in hand, asking others to join him. I occasionally hike with a 5-decade Rosary, but it's awkward to use while running, cycling, or at the gym.

A more practical option in such cases is to use a Rosary bracelet, Rosary ring, or decade Rosary. They're available at most Catholic bookstores or online. These single-decade Rosaries usually consist of a crucifix, one bead or knot for the Our Father and 10 Hail Mary beads or knots. They are a type of shortcut to help keep track of the prayers. I have found a small cord-style, single-decade Rosary with knots rather than beads to be the perfect solution for running workouts. Rosary rings or finger Rosaries are also easy to carry. Request a free finger Rosary at this site: **www.fingerrosaries.com**

A simple method is to use your fingers to count the prayers. To avoid confusion, always start the decade with the same hand and same finger/thumb so you'll know your "place". This is the only way that I can safely pray a Rosary while I'm cycling.

Swimming is a bit trickier. I count how many Hail Mary's I can pray during a lap of the pool at a given pace and stroke, then calculate how many laps or lengths I need to swim to complete ten Hail Mary's. Perhaps you'll come up with something more creative.

At the gym, I use a single-decade Rosary or the number buttons on the cardio machines to keep track of the prayers. Most machines have a keypad with the numbers 1-10 on the display panel. I focus on each number in turn while meditating on the mystery.

I do have to admit that my MP-3 player is my favorite tool for praying the Rosary during exercise. I downloaded a Rosary CD with background music, and this really frees me to meditate on the mysteries as I exercise. One caveat: Do not use headphones if you are exercising in dangerous situations or supervising young children while you exercise.

Try to limit distractions during your workouts with the Rosary. If you are exercising in an environment that is not conducive to meditative prayer, you may want to eliminate the inclusion of prayer that day.

You'll inevitably lose track of the prayers or even forget which mystery you should be contemplating. Keep working on this skill, but don't despair. This is my solution: All extra prayers are offered for the Souls in Purgatory, and I ask my guardian angel to finish any prayers that I forgot.

Role Models *"[Show] yourselves as a model of good deeds in every respect, with integrity in your teaching, dignity, and sound speech that cannot be criticized."* (Titus 2:7-8)

It's always helpful to find a role model for inspiration when beginning a new activity or undertaking. Although there are many popes, saints and other holy people who are both athletic and spiritual, I've chosen a few who are especially relevant to "Rosary athletes".

St. Aybert, who lived in the 12th century, was one of the earliest documented practitioners of a type of Rosary workout. He recited 150 Ave Marias (the earliest version of the Hail Mary) every day while genuflecting and prostrating himself on the floor.

St. Dominic (1172-1221) and **St. Louis de Montfort** (1673-1716) are responsible for spreading a worldwide devotion to the Rosary and the Blessed Mother. Both saints were strong, athletic young men who walked thousands of miles throughout Europe while preaching about the Rosary.

A more contemporary role model, especially for young people, is **Blessed Pier Giorgio Frassati** (1901-1925), a handsome young Italian athlete with a lifelong devotion to the Rosary. He was an avid runner, swimmer, cyclist, hiker, equestrian, skater, and skier who found the energy and strength for his passions through daily reception of the Holy Eucharist. Pier Giorgio is a shining example of a modern Catholic youth who continues to influence young athletes today. There are many websites devoted to him.

The late **Pope John Paul II** was beloved by many and well-known as a promoter of peace, but few are aware that he was a very gifted athlete. He played soccer, skied, cycled, swam and conquered many arduous Alpine peaks. He viewed exercise in the great outdoors as an opportunity for meditation and spiritual development.

Women can find a source of inspiration in **St. Gianna Molla** (1822-1962). She was an athlete, a pediatrician and an avid skier. She made the ultimate sacrifice by giving her life for one of her children by choosing to die during childbirth rather than abort her baby.

Another source of inspiration for women of all ages can be found in two Catholic athletes who are still competing today: Rebecca Dussault and Sister Madonna Buder. **Rebecca Dussault** is an Olympic cross-country skier who also participates in many other sports. She put her athletic goals and dreams on hold to raise her children and to help her husband fight a near-deadly disease. She turns to Blessed Pier Giorgio Frassati as a role model as she aspires to "live heroic virtue and become a saint."

Sister Madonna Buder discovered the benefits of exercise fairly late in life, at age 49, when a priest recommended that she take up running to aid in her meditation. She enjoyed exercise so much that she began to compete in triathlons. Today she holds the title of the "World's Oldest Female Triathlete." She is a regular competitor in the Hawaii Ironman Triathlon, a grueling race which requires a 2.4-mile ocean swim, 112 miles of cycling and a marathon run (26.2 miles). Sister Buder does not let her athletic training interfere with good works. She dedicates each competition to someone in need, is active in her religious community and ministers to prisoners.

You'll find a diverse group of Catholic athletes – male and female, young and old, professional and amateur – to inspire you at Catholic Athletes for Christ:
www.catholicathletesforchrist.com

"Those who do not find time for exercise will have to find time for illness." - Earl of Derby

Part V:

The Workouts

Beginner

Intermediate

Advanced

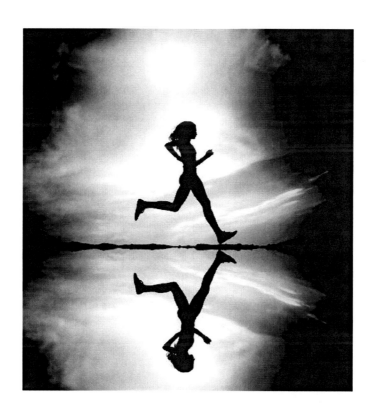

The Beginner Series

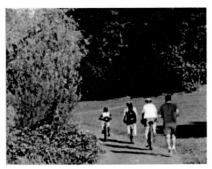

As a Beginner, you are building a very important foundation for the integration of prayer and exercise. You certainly would not build a house on a foundation of sand. In the same way, you should not continue to the Intermediate and Advanced Series until you have mastered the skill of praying and meditating on the Rosary while exercising at the same time. To advance without attaining proficiency in these areas could result in an injury or reduce your ability to focus on meditation.

Jesus makes a similar comparison with the Word of God:

"Everyone who listens to these words of mine and acts on them will be like a wise man who built his house on rock. The rain fell, the floods came, and the winds blew and buffeted the house. But it did not collapse; it had been set solidly on rock. And everyone who listens to these words of mine but does not act on them will be like a fool who built his house on sand. The rain fell, the floods came, and the winds blew and buffeted the house. And it collapsed and was completely ruined." (Matthew 7: 24-27)

The Beginner Series is the "foundation of rock" upon which you will build your physical <u>and</u> spiritual fitness. Enjoy these early workouts for their simplicity as The Rosary Workout™ prepares you for significant and life-changing achievements.

Perseverance:

Unfortunately, beginners are the most likely to quit a new program. Jesus addresses this problem in the Parable of the Sower:

"The seed sown on rocky ground is the one who hears the Word and receives it at once with joy. But he has no root and lasts only for a time. When some tribulation or persecution comes because of the Word, he immediately falls away." (Matthew 13: 20-21)

If you experience difficulty with Beginner Series workouts or with praying the Rosary, refer to the sections on Discipline and Setbacks. Keep praying for assistance.

Beginner Series Goals:

There are three primary goals in the Beginner Series:

1. Establish a habit of regular exercise
2. Establish a habit of regular Rosary prayer
3. Learn to integrate prayer, exercise and meditation

The workouts are sub-divided into three levels: **Angel**, **Archangel** and **Principality**, which include specific, parallel goals for physical and spiritual growth and habit formation. I have included modifications throughout this series for readers who may be more experienced with exercise or Rosary prayer.

Each level begins with a prayer to the particular choir of angels to which the level is dedicated. Next, you'll find an overview and a list of specific goals. Then the actual workouts are described, grouped by weeks. Rosary graphics are included to help you understand how the workout corresponds to the Rosary prayers. All levels conclude with a "homework" assignment as an added challenge.

If you are at an intermediate or advanced level in terms of exercise and/or praying the Rosary, you are likely still a beginner in terms of integrating the two. Readers of all fitness abilities should complete the Archangel Level to learn the important skill of praying and meditating while exercising. This is a skill which requires patience and plenty of practice.

Before you lace up your shoes, take a few minutes to read through the workouts for the level that best suits your current fitness state. It's important that you understand the physical and spiritual goals as well as the specifics of each workout.

Angel Level Workouts: First Beginner Level (4 weeks)

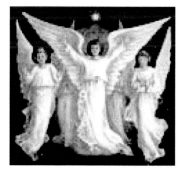

Prayer to the **Choir of Angels**:

By the intercession of St. Michael and the celestial Choir of Angels may the Lord grant us to be protected by them in this mortal life and conducted in the life to come to Heaven. Amen.

-From the Chaplet of St. Michael the Archangel

Pray to the Choir of Angels and your own guardian angel to ask their assistance in completing this level.

Angel Level Summary and Goals:

The Angel Level is all about habit formation — establishing a habit of regular exercise and regular Rosary prayer. You should keep these two goals in mind when scheduling your workouts. Please don't try to do any extra workouts as this gradual and gentle approach is designed to prevent injury and a sense of being overwhelmed.

This level is best suited for those who have not exercised in a long time or who have never exercised. It's also appropriate for the elderly, children and teens, pregnant and post-partum women or those recovering from a recent illness or injury. If you fall into one of the above categories, please consult your doctor before exercising to determine any modifications or limitations.

The Angel Level is also designed for those who have not memorized all the Rosary prayers and the 20 mysteries. If you exercise regularly, then simply modify the workouts to fit your current fitness level as you work on memorizing the prayers and mysteries. Move to the next level when you have completed the memorization requirements.

Skip this level if you exercise regularly (2-3 days each week for at least 20 minutes per workout) AND you are familiar with the Rosary prayers and all 20 mysteries.

Angel Level Goals:

1. Establish a habit of regular exercise and regular Rosary prayer

2. Memorize the Rosary prayers and the titles of all 20 mysteries

After completing the Angel Level you should be able to:

1. Pray a full Rosary from memory and recite the titles of all 20 mysteries

2. Exercise continuously for at least 20 minutes

Spiritual Components for the Angel Level:

Beginners in Mary's School of the Rosary: Memorize the basic prayers of the Rosary and the titles of the 20 mysteries. Refer to Appendix A-E for a tutorial on the Rosary.

Intermediate and advanced students of Mary's School: If you are very familiar with the Rosary and pray it often but are a beginner to exercise, perhaps you can memorize a few new prayers or passages from Scripture.

Exercise Components for the Angel Level:

Frequency: 2 days per week

Duration: 9-20 minutes per workout (including warm-up and cool-down)

Note: The timing for each segment of the workout is included as a guideline. Your personal time for the warm-up, workout and cool-down may vary as you learn and memorize the prayers and mysteries of the Rosary. By the end of the Angel Level, you should be able to pray a five-decade Rosary in approximately 20 minutes.

Intensity:

Warm-up and cool-down: Very Easy to Easy (2-3 on RPE scale)

Base pace: Easy to Moderate (3-4 on the RPE scale)

Mode: Any type of rhythmic aerobic exercise (walking, biking, etc.). Use the same mode of exercise for all workouts in this level.

Angel Level Warm-up: The Angel Level warm-up is the same throughout all the workouts in this level and is therefore listed only once. There are two components to the warm-up:

Spiritual warm-up: Before you begin the physical portion of the warm-up, you should first "warm-up" spiritually with a short prayer to the Holy Spirit, your patron saint or the Blessed Mother asking for help in learning to pray the Rosary as you exercise. Decide on a Rosary intention based on your own needs or those of others.

Physical warm-up: The physical warm-up will take you through the first part of the Rosary using the crucifix and the first four beads on the pendant chain. Begin the warm-up at an RPE of 2-3 while you pray the Apostles' Creed, Our Father, 3 Hail Mary's, Glory Be, and Fatima Prayer. These prayers should take approximately 3 minutes. (If this takes you more time as you learn the prayers and mysteries of the Rosary, feel free to shorten the rest of the planned workout based on your fitness level or time constraints.) You are ready to begin your workout with the first decade of the Rosary.

Angel Level Cool-down: The Angel Level cool-down is also the same throughout all the workouts in this level and is therefore listed only once. Slow your pace to an RPE of 2-3 as you pray a decade of the Rosary and the Hail Holy Queen (see note below), which is prayed on the medal that connects the circular portion of the Rosary. These prayers should take approximately 3-4 minutes. If this takes you more time as you learn the prayers and mysteries of the Rosary, feel free to shorten the length of the cool-down, based on your fitness level.

Note: You'll end the workouts with the Hail Holy Queen, even if you did not complete all five decades of the Rosary so that you can learn this prayer through frequent recitation.

Stretch: If time allows after your workout, take a few minutes to stretch the major muscle groups you worked during exercise. This is a good time to finish the Rosary prayers. If you don't have time to stretch, try to fit in a stretching session later in the day or at least 2-3 times each week.

Angel Level Week 1

Spiritual Component: Begin working toward the Angel Level goal of memorizing the Rosary prayers. This week you'll memorize the titles of the five Joyful Mysteries:

1. The Annunciation
2. The Visitation
3. The Nativity (or Birth of Jesus)
4. The Presentation
5. The Finding of the Child Jesus in the Temple

Workout 1 (9-13 minutes total time):

Focus: In the Angel Level, the focus is on gradually increasing exercise duration as you progress to praying a full Rosary during exercise. You will begin with a goal of 1-2 decades of the Rosary. A decade consists of announcing the mystery, praying the Our Father, 10 Hail Mary's, Glory Be and Fatima Prayer. The first decade begins on the pendant chain on the fifth bead with the announcement of the first mystery and the Our Father. It continues with the first group of 10 Hail Mary's on the circular chain.

Don't try to do too much too soon. If you become overly fatigued or start breathing heavily, slow down or stop and catch your breath. The suggested workouts are simply goals, not requirements. Remember, the workouts of the Angel Level promote habit formation, not competition or trying to get back in shape in one week!

Note: Since you won't pray the entire Rosary during your workout, try to find time to finish it later, perhaps while you're stretching.

Warm up: Refer to the **Angel Level Warm-up** instructions at the beginning of this section (approximately 3 minutes).

Workout: After the warm-up, increase intensity slightly to your base pace (RPE of 3-4), and pray one or two decades of the Rosary. Pray the Joyful Mysteries today to help with your memorization. The following is a graphic representation of this workout.

Cool-down/Stretch: Refer to the **Angel Level Cool-down** at the beginning of this section (3-4 minutes).

Journal entry: Log the workout in your journal. Add plenty of details.

Workout 2 (9-13 minutes total time):

Repeat Workout 1. Try to schedule at least 1-2 days of rest between workouts.

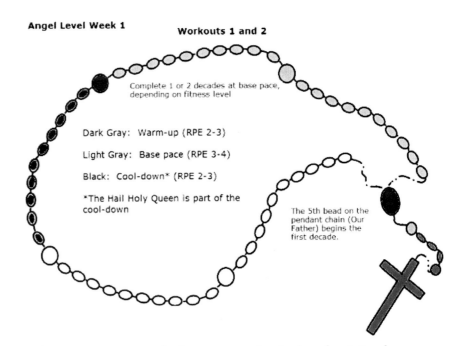

Angel Level Week 1

Workouts 1 and 2

Complete 1 or 2 decades at base pace, depending on fitness level

Dark Gray: Warm-up (RPE 2-3)

Light Gray: Base pace (RPE 3-4)

Black: Cool-down* (RPE 2-3)

*The Hail Holy Queen is part of the cool-down

The 5th bead on the pendant chain (Our Father) begins the first decade.

Great work! You've taken an important step on the journey to physical and spiritual fitness.

<u>Spiritual Component:</u>   Continue working toward the Angel Level goal of memorizing the Rosary prayers. This week you'll memorize the titles of the five Luminous Mysteries:

1. The Baptism of Jesus
2. The Wedding Feast at Cana
3. The Proclamation of the Kingdom
4. The Transfiguration
5. The Institution of the Eucharist

Workout 1 (12-16 minutes total time):

Focus: This week you will increase exercise duration by adding one more decade to your workout. If an additional decade is too much, try to at least add an Our Father and 1-5 Hail Mary's.

Keep in mind that you are just trying to exercise slightly longer than last week, even if it's just a minute or two. If you worked too hard last week and feel sore or discouraged, then back off a bit this week. This program allows for all the time you need to meet the Angel Level goals.

<u>Note:</u> Since you won't pray the entire Rosary during your workout, try to find time to finish it later, perhaps while you're stretching.

Warm up: Refer to the **Angel Level Warm-up** instructions at the beginning of this section (approximately 3 minutes)

Workout: After the warm-up, increase intensity to your base pace (RPE of 3-4), and pray two to three decades of the Rosary. Pray the Luminous Mysteries today to help with your memorization. A graphic representation of this workout can be found on the next page.

Cool-down/Stretch: Refer to the **Angel Level Cool-down** at the beginning of this section (3-4 minutes).

Journal entry: Log your workout in your journal.

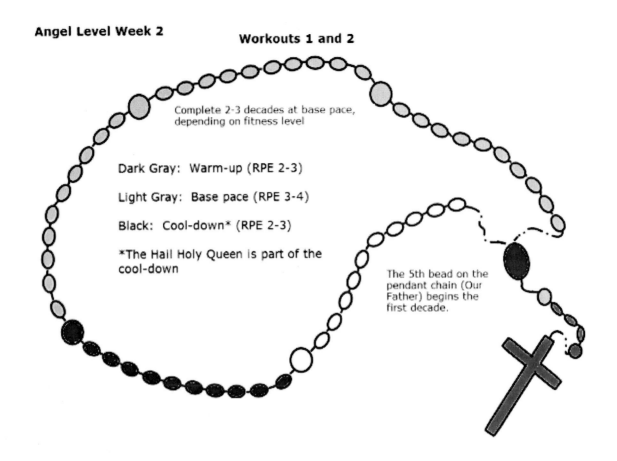

Angel Level Week 2

Workouts 1 and 2

Complete 2-3 decades at base pace, depending on fitness level

Dark Gray: Warm-up (RPE 2-3)

Light Gray: Base pace (RPE 3-4)

Black: Cool-down* (RPE 2-3)

*The Hail Holy Queen is part of the cool-down

The 5th bead on the pendant chain (Our Father) begins the first decade.

Workout 2 (12-16 minutes total time):

Repeat Workout 1. Allow at least one or two days of rest between workouts.

Congratulations! You're halfway through the Angel Level. Keep up the good work.

"You shall obtain all you ask of me by the recitation of the Rosary." - Our Lady to Blessed Alan de la Roche

<u>Spiritual Component:</u>   Continue working toward the Angel Level goal of memorizing the Rosary prayers. This week you'll memorize the titles of the five Sorrowful Mysteries:

1. The Agony in the Garden
2. The Scourging at the Pillar
3. The Crowning of Thorns
4. The Carrying of the Cross
5. The Crucifixion

Workout 1 (15-19 minutes total time):

Focus: This week you will add an additional decade to your workout. Keep in mind that you are just trying to exercise slightly longer than last week, even if it's just a minute or two. If you worked too hard last week and feel sore or discouraged, then back off a bit this week. Don't despair if you are only able to pray a decade or two. This program allows for all the time you need to meet the Angel Level goals.

Workout: Following the **Angel Level Warm-up**, increase intensity to your base pace (RPE of 3-4), and pray three to four decades of the Rosary. Finish with the **Angel Level Cool-down**. Pray the Sorrowful Mysteries today to help with your memorization. A graphic representation of this workout can be found on the next page.

Journal entry: Log your workout in your journal.

Workout 2 (15-19 minutes total time):

Repeat Workout 1. Allow at least one or two days of rest between workouts.

Keep it up! Just one more week left to reach your first milestone in The Rosary Workout™.

"If you persevere in reciting the Rosary, this will be a most probable sign of your eternal salvation." - Blessed Alan de la Roche

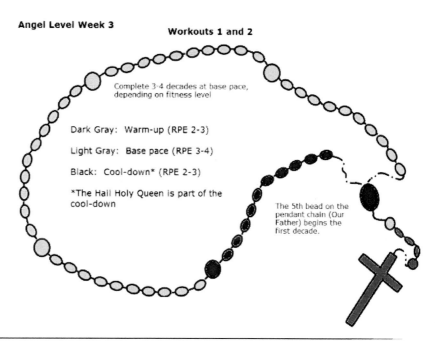

Angel Level Week 3

Workouts 1 and 2

Complete 3-4 decades at base pace, depending on fitness level

Dark Gray: Warm-up (RPE 2-3)

Light Gray: Base pace (RPE 3-4)

Black: Cool-down* (RPE 2-3)

*The Hail Holy Queen is part of the cool-down

The 5th bead on the pendant chain (Our Father) begins the first decade.

Spiritual Component: By the end of this week, you should reach the Angel Level goal of memorizing all the Rosary prayers.   You'll also memorize the titles of the five Glorious Mysteries:

1. The Resurrection
2. The Ascension
3. The Descent of the Holy Spirit
4. The Assumption
5. The Coronation (Crowning of Mary as Queen of Heaven and Earth)

Workout 1 (18-20 minutes total time):

Focus: The goal for this week is to pray a five-decade Rosary during exercise.   The total workout should last approximately 18-20 minutes, including warm-up and cool-down.   If it takes you significantly more time to pray the Rosary, then limit the total workout duration to 20 minutes. (Finish praying the Rosary during your stretching session or later in the day.)   If you are not able to exercise for 20 minutes, try to add an additional decade or part of a decade to your previous workout.

Workout: Following the **Angel Level Warm-up**, increase intensity to your base pace (RPE of 3-4), and pray four decades of the Rosary.   Transition to the **Angel Level Cool-down** at the beginning of the 5th decade.   Pray the Glorious Mysteries today to help with your memorization.   A graphic representation of this workout can be found on the next page.

Journal entry: Log your workout in your journal.

Workout 2 (18-20 minutes total time):

Repeat Workout 1.   Allow at least one or two days of rest between workouts.

Note: If you can't exercise continuously for 20 minutes by the end of this week, keep building on your current workout level every week until you reach 20 minutes.   Don't be discouraged if this takes some time.   For motivation, look back over your journal entries to see how far you've come.

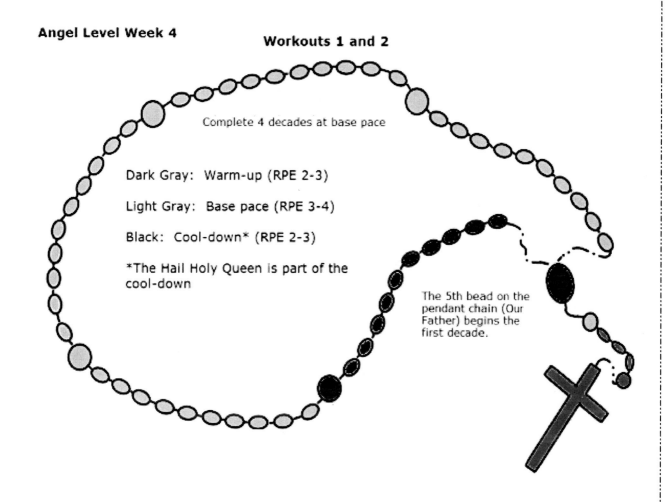

Angel Level Week 4

Workouts 1 and 2

Complete 4 decades at base pace

Dark Gray: Warm-up (RPE 2-3)

Light Gray: Base pace (RPE 3-4)

Black: Cool-down* (RPE 2-3)

*The Hail Holy Queen is part of the cool-down

The 5th bead on the pendant chain (Our Father) begins the first decade.

Congratulations! You have completed the Angel Level of The Rosary Workout™. You've memorized the prayers and mysteries of the Rosary, and you've begun an important habit of regular Rosary prayer. Perhaps you're experiencing a renewal in your faith. You're also starting to notice some of the benefits of regular exercise. You have more energy, you sleep more soundly and your sense of self-esteem has increased with the completion of four weeks of regular exercise.

Angel Level Graduation Requirements

You are ready to progress to the Archangel Level if you have met the following conditions:

1. You can pray a complete Rosary from memory while exercising and can recite the titles of all 20 mysteries.
2. You have exercised 2 days each week for 4 continuous weeks.
3. You are able to exercise continuously for at least 20 minutes.
4. If you have not met the three conditions above, consider extra study and/or workouts before you progress to the Archangel Level. If you are not confident about your ability to pray the Rosary and recall all 20 mysteries, then keep practicing. If you struggle with the workouts, continue building on the progress you've made so far until you are able to meet the frequency and duration goals above.
5. Reward yourself for reaching your goal.
6. Don't forget to pray to the Choir of Angels (and any saints to whom you prayed for intercession) to thank them for their assistance in helping you complete this level.

Angel Level Completion Assignments:

There are two "homework" assignments, one for the body and one for the soul, at the end of each level. They encourage you to explore other aspects of faith and fitness outside the scope of The Rosary Workout™. These assignments are meant to challenge and not to overwhelm you. If the homework at this level is not feasible, take a look at the assignments for other levels. If you must skip the assignments, then revisit them later in the program.

For the Soul: It has been at least a month since you began this program, so it's time to visit the confessional. Regular reception of this important sacrament is essential to your spiritual health.

Additionally, take at least 10 minutes sometime this week to visit the Blessed Sacrament. If you're not familiar with this custom, it is the practice of praying before the Tabernacle in a Catholic church. The location of the Tabernacle is marked by a red light or lamp, known as the sanctuary lamp, indicating that Jesus is present in the Eucharist when it is lit. In some Catholic churches, the Tabernacle is directly behind the altar or located to one side in the main church. Other churches have a separate Blessed Sacrament Chapel. If you're not sure, call the parish office. In fact, it's a good idea to call to determine if the church will be open at the time of your planned visit.

During your visit, thank the Blessed Mother and her Divine Son for the strength and perseverance to make it through the Angel Level.

Extra Credit: Make time to visit the Blessed Sacrament at least once a week. If you can't find time during the week, try to arrive at Sunday Mass a few minutes early or stay after Mass to make your visit. The sick, homebound or those in remote areas can visit the Blessed Sacrament online: **www.savior.org** (Even if you're not sick or homebound, this site is worth checking out.)

Some parishes offer Eucharistic Adoration or even Perpetual Adoration, when the Blessed Sacrament is exposed on the altar in a beautiful gold receptacle called a monstrance. Parish members sign up for blocks of time during Eucharistic Adoration to ensure that the Blessed Sacrament is never unattended.

For the Body: Make a commitment to add one fruit or vegetable to your diet, every day from now on. Try something new like kiwi, turnips, or cauliflower. Search your cookbook collection, the local library or the internet for a recipe that includes the new fruit or vegetable.

Archangel Level Workouts: Second Beginner Level (4 weeks)

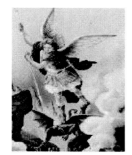

Prayer to the **Choir of Archangels:**

By the intercession of St. Michael and the celestial Choir of Archangels may the Lord give us perseverance in faith and in all good works in order that we may attain the glory of Heaven. Amen.
-From the Chaplet of St. Michael the Archangel

Say a prayer to the Choir of Archangels and your own guardian angel to ask their assistance in completing this level.

Archangel Level Summary and Goals:

The Archangel Level builds on the foundation of the Angel Level. You have established a habit of regular workouts and are familiar with the Rosary prayers and mysteries. Now you're ready to integrate exercise and meditation.

Archangels are the most important angels in the Bible.   Likewise, the Archangel Level is the most important level in The Rosary Workout™ because it is essential that you learn how to use the rhythm of exercise in harmony with the rhythm of the repeated Hail Mary's to attain a meditative state.   Rhythmic cardiovascular exercise at a fairly comfortable pace serves to open the mind to clearer thought and a heightened awareness. The workouts will aid you in directing this clarity of mind toward meditative prayer.

Combining exercise and Rosary meditation is challenging and requires practice to master. The workouts of the Archangel Level are deliberately basic and repetitive to facilitate meditation. It's natural and expected that you will get distracted and struggle with this combination in the beginning. Persevere, pray for help, and remember that you're building a "foundation of rock".

Readers of all fitness abilities should complete the Archangel Level to learn the important skill of praying and meditating while exercising. Intermediate and advanced exercisers can modify the suggested workout parameters based on their current fitness.

The Archangel Level is unique as it is subdivided into two programs. Program 1 gradually increases the frequency of workouts to three days per week while keeping the workout duration at 20 minutes. Program 2 gradually increases the workout duration to 30 minutes while maintaining the frequency at two days per week. The dual options offer a choice to accommodate those who may have limited time to exercise but still want to improve fitness.

Archangel Level Goals:

1. Continue building a habit of regular exercise and regular Rosary prayer, but add the challenge of an extra day or additional time.

2. Integrate prayer and exercise by focusing on meditation

3. Read and study passages from the Bible that pertain to each mystery in order to create a mental picture of each event.

After completing the Archangel Level you should be able to:

1. Meditate on the Rosary mysteries during exercise

2. Exercise twice a week for 30 minutes **or** three times a week for 20 minutes

3. Be familiar with the Biblical references to each mystery of the Rosary

Spiritual Components for the Archangel Level:

Beginners in Mary's School of the Rosary: Each week you will read a section of the Bible that describes one of the four sets of mysteries. These readings will help you form a mental picture on which to focus meditation. Try to memorize a verse or two to remind you of the reading. Week 1 will include the Joyful Mysteries, Week 2 the Luminous Mysteries, Week 3 the Sorrowful Mysteries and Week 4 the Glorious Mysteries.

Intermediate and advanced students in Mary's School of the Rosary: Although you are probably very familiar with the Rosary mysteries, the integration of exercise, prayer and meditation may be challenging. During the workouts, allow the exercise rhythm to help focus your mind on the mysteries, drawing on your past study to experience a new state of meditative prayer. The spiritual assignments in this level are geared toward those new to Rosary meditation, so feel free to modify them.

A suggestion is to re-read the Bible references to each mystery from a new perspective by comparing them in different translations of Catholic Bibles. Online versions:

New American Catholic Bible: **www.usccb.org/nab/bible**
Douay-Rheims Catholic Bible: **www.drbo.org**
Revised Standard Version (RSV) Catholic Edition:
www.ewtn.com/devotionals/biblesearch.asp

Exercise Components for the Archangel Level:

Frequency: Increase to 3 days each week (Program 1) **OR** continue frequency at 2 days per week (Program 2)

Duration: Maintain at 20 minutes (Program 1) **OR** increase to 30 minutes (Program 2)

Note: I am making the assumption that you can pray a five-decade Rosary in 18-20 minutes. If it takes you significantly more time to pray the Rosary, then limit the total workout time to 20 minutes. (Finish praying the Rosary during your stretching session or later in the day.)

Intensity:

Warm-up and cool-down: Very Easy to Easy (2-3 on RPE scale)

Base pace: Easy to Moderate (3-4 on the RPE scale)

Note: Experienced exercisers can adjust the RPE, duration and frequency as needed.

Mode: Any type of rhythmic aerobic exercise (walking, biking, etc.) Use the same mode of exercise that you used in the Angel Level, but you should vary your routine occasionally. For instance if you walked the same route every day in the Angel Level, try a different route. If you were exercising inside, try going outside if weather permits.

Archangel Level Warm-up: The Archangel Level warm-up is the same throughout all the workouts in this level and is therefore listed only once.

Spiritual warm-up: Before you begin the physical portion of the warm-up, you should first "warm-up" spiritually with a short prayer to the Holy Spirit, your patron saint or the Blessed Mother asking for help in meditating on each mystery of the Rosary as you exercise. Decide on a Rosary intention based on your own needs or those of others.

Physical warm-up: Begin exercise at an RPE of 2-3 while you pray the Apostles' Creed, Our Father, 3 Hail Mary's, Glory Be, and Fatima Prayer. These prayers should take approximately 3 minutes. You are ready to begin your workout with the first decade of the Rosary.

Archangel Level Cool-down: The Archangel Level cool-down is also the same throughout all the workouts in this level. Slow your pace to an RPE of 2-3 as you pray the 5th decade of the Rosary and the Hail Holy Queen, which is prayed on the medal that connects the circular portion of the Rosary (approximately 3-4 minutes). If you are able to finish the Rosary before the cool-down period, then use this time to reflect on the mysteries or enjoy your surroundings and the great feeling of accomplishment in finishing your workout.

Stretch: If time allows after your workout, take a few minutes to stretch the major muscle groups you worked during exercise. If you don't have time to stretch, try to fit in a stretching session later in the day or at least 2-3 times each week.

Archangel Level (Program 1) Week 1
Increasing frequency to 3 days per week

Note: If you prefer to keep the frequency at two days per week while increasing duration, then skip to **Archangel Level Program 2**

Spiritual Component: Read the Bible references for each of the **Joyful Mysteries**. (See Appendix C) If you focus on the readings for one mystery a day, the time commitment is just a few minutes each day for five days this week.

Workout 1 (20 minutes total time):

Focus: Reflect on the Joyful Mysteries today to reinforce this week's Bible readings. Try to establish a consistent rhythm during the main workout to facilitate prayerful meditation.

Workout: After the **Archangel Level warm-up**, increase intensity to an RPE of 3-4. This is your "**base pace**" and represents an intensity you can comfortably maintain for 15-20 minutes. Pray the first four decades of the Rosary. Transition to the **Archangel Level cool-down** during the 5th decade. Total workout time is 20 minutes, including warm-up and cool-down.

Journal entry: Log your workout in your journal.

"... The Holy Rosary is not a pious practice banished to the past, like prayers of other times thought of with nostalgia. Instead, the Rosary is experiencing a new Springtime. Without a doubt, this is one of the most eloquent signs of love that the young generation nourish for Jesus and His Mother, Mary. In the current world, so dispersive, this prayer helps to put Christ at the centre, as the Virgin did, who meditated within all that was said about her Son, and also what He did and said. When reciting the Rosary, the important and meaningful moments of salvation history are relived. The various steps of Christ's mission are traced. With Mary the heart is oriented toward the mystery of Jesus. Christ is put at the centre of our life, of our time, of our city, through the contemplation and meditation of His holy mysteries of joy, light, sorrow and glory. May Mary help us to welcome within ourselves the grace emanating from these mysteries, so that through us we can "water" society, beginning with our daily relationships, and purifying them from so many negative forces, thus opening them to the newness of God. The Rosary, when it is prayed in an authentic way, not mechanical and superficial but profoundly, it brings, in fact, peace and reconciliation. It contains within itself the healing power of the Most Holy Name of Jesus, invoked with faith and love at the centre of each "Hail Mary". - Pope Benedict XVI, Address to the Basilica of St. Mary Major, 3 May 2008

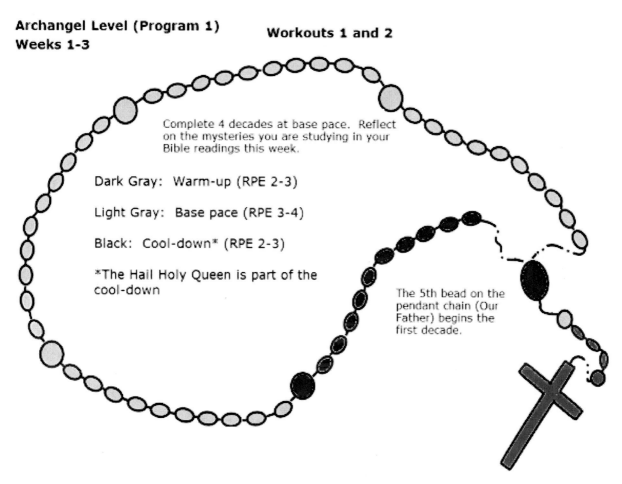

Archangel Level (Program 1)
Weeks 1-3

Workouts 1 and 2

Complete 4 decades at base pace. Reflect on the mysteries you are studying in your Bible readings this week.

Dark Gray: Warm-up (RPE 2-3)

Light Gray: Base pace (RPE 3-4)

Black: Cool-down* (RPE 2-3)

*The Hail Holy Queen is part of the cool-down

The 5th bead on the pendant chain (Our Father) begins the first decade.

<u>Note:</u> Refer to this graphic for Weeks 1-3, Workouts 1 and 2

Workout 2 (20 minutes total time):

Repeat Workout 1. Try to allow at least one day of rest between workouts.

Workout 3 (9-13 minutes total time):

Focus: Since this is the first day of increasing frequency to 3 days per week, you should keep this workout fairly short. Continue to reflect on the Joyful Mysteries.

Workout: After the **Archangel Level warm-up**, increase intensity to your base pace (RPE of 3-4), and pray one or two decades of the Rosary (about 3-6 minutes). Transition to the **Archangel Level cool-down**.

Journal entry: Log your workout in your journal.

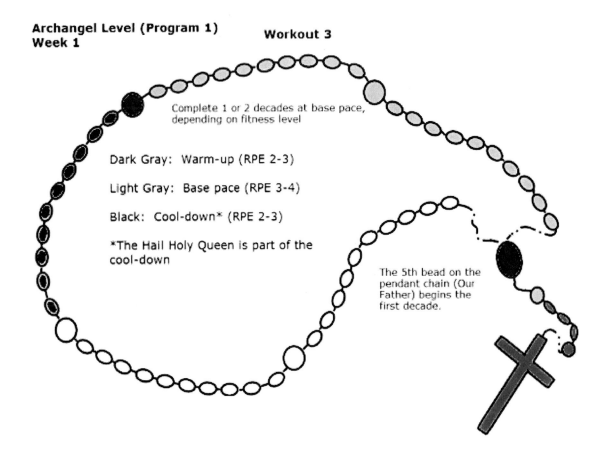

Archangel Level (Program 1)
Week 1

Workout 3

Complete 1 or 2 decades at base pace, depending on fitness level

Dark Gray: Warm-up (RPE 2-3)

Light Gray: Base pace (RPE 3-4)

Black: Cool-down* (RPE 2-3)

*The Hail Holy Queen is part of the cool-down

The 5th bead on the pendant chain (Our Father) begins the first decade.

Great work this week! You are receiving so many graces through your regular Rosary prayer.

Blessing of the Rosary: Those who weep find happiness.

<u>Spiritual Component</u>: Read the Bible references for the **Luminous Mysteries** (Appendix C). If you focus on the readings for one mystery a day, the time commitment is just a few minutes each day for five days this week.

Workout 1 (20 minutes total time):

<u>Focus:</u> Reflect on the Luminous Mysteries today to reinforce this week's Bible readings. As you exercise, try to create a mental picture of each mystery to aid in meditation.

<u>Workout:</u> After the **Archangel Level warm-up**, increase intensity to your base pace (RPE of 3-4), and pray four decades of the Rosary. Transition to the **Archangel Level cool-down** at the beginning of the 5th decade as you finish the Rosary. Total workout time should be about 20 minutes, including warm-up and cool-down.

<u>Journal entry</u>: Log your workout in your journal.

Workout 2 (20 minutes total time):

Repeat Workout 1. Try to allow at least one day of rest between workouts.

Workout 3 (12-16 minutes total time):

<u>Focus:</u> This is your second week of increasing frequency of workouts. Your goal today is to try to exercise a little longer than you did last week. (Check your journal to determine how long you exercised during Workout 3 last week, and add an additional decade or part of a decade.) Continue to reflect on the Luminous Mysteries.

<u>Workout:</u> After the **Archangel Level warm-up**, increase intensity to your base pace (RPE of 3-4), and pray two or three decades of the Rosary (about 6-9 minutes). Transition to the **Archangel Level cool-down**.

<u>Journal entry</u>: Log your workout in your journal.

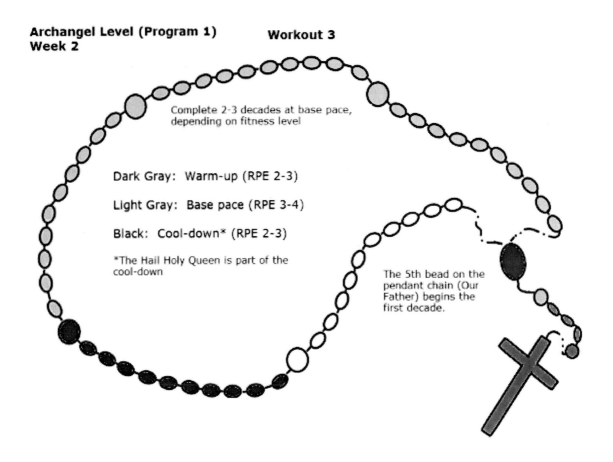

Archangel Level (Program 1) Week 2   **Workout 3**

Complete 2-3 decades at base pace, depending on fitness level

Dark Gray: Warm-up (RPE 2-3)

Light Gray: Base pace (RPE 3-4)

Black: Cool-down* (RPE 2-3)

*The Hail Holy Queen is part of the cool-down

The 5th bead on the pendant chain (Our Father) begins the first decade.

Well done! In addition to receiving the spiritual benefits and blessings of regular Rosary prayer, you're also reducing the risk of many life-threatening diseases such as diabetes, cancer, high blood pressure and heart disease.

<u>Spiritual Component</u>:   Read the Bible references for the **Sorrowful Mysteries** (Refer to Appendix C).

Workout 1 (20 minutes total time):

Focus: Reflect on the Sorrowful Mysteries today. After establishing a comfortable rhythm at your base pace, concentrate on the scene of each mystery. Imagine yourself as an observer, drawing on details from this week's Bible readings.

Workout: After the **Archangel Level warm-up**, increase intensity to your base pace (RPE of 3-4), and pray four decades of the Rosary. Transition to the **Archangel Level cool-down** at the beginning of the 5th decade and finish the Rosary.

Journal entry: Log your workout in your journal.

Workout 2 (20 minutes total time):

Repeat Workout 1. Allow at least one day of rest between workouts.

Workout 3 (20 minutes total time):

Focus: By now, you should be able to complete a Rosary during 20 minutes of continuous exercise, three days each week. If this is too challenging, keep adding time to this third workout each week until you reach the goal of 20 minutes. Reflect on the Sorrowful Mysteries today.

Workout: After the **Archangel Level warm-up**, increase intensity to your base pace (RPE of 3-4), and pray four decades of the Rosary. Transition to the **Archangel Level cool-down** at the beginning of the 5th decade and finish the Rosary.   Total workout time should be about 20 minutes, including warm-up and cool-down.

Journal entry: Log your workout in your journal.

Mary promised: Whoever shall recite the Rosary devoutly, applying themselves to the consideration of its Sacred Mysteries, shall never be conquered by misfortune. God will not chastise them in His justice, they shall not perish by an unprovided death; if they are just, they shall remain in the grace of God, and become worthy of eternal life.

<u>Spiritual Component</u>: Read the Bible references for the **Glorious Mysteries** (Appendix C).

Workout 1 (20 minutes total time):

Focus: Reflect on the Glorious Mysteries, based on your readings from the Bible. During your cool-down, think of a good deed that you can do for someone today.

Workout: After the **Archangel Level warm-up**, increase intensity to base pace (RPE of 3-4), and pray four decades of the Rosary. Transition to the **Archangel Level cool-down** at the beginning of the 5th decade. Total time is 20 minutes, including warm-up and cool-down.

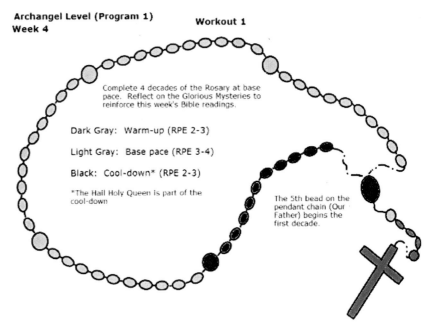

Archangel Level (Program 1) Week 4

Workout 1

Complete 4 decades of the Rosary at base pace. Reflect on the Glorious Mysteries to reinforce this week's Bible readings.

Dark Gray: Warm-up (RPE 2-3)

Light Gray: Base pace (RPE 3-4)

Black: Cool-down* (RPE 2-3)

*The Hail Holy Queen is part of the cool-down

The 5th bead on the pendant chain (Our Father) begins the first decade.

Journal entry: Log your workout in your journal.

Workout 2 (20 minutes total time):

Focus: Today's workout is easier than usual. An easy workout now and then provides a physical and mental break. To add variety, try a different mode of exercise or invite a friend or family member to accompany you. If you pray the Rosary, take turns reciting the prayers. The traditional method is for one person to say the first half of each prayer and the other(s) to finish it. You may need to decrease the RPE to allow for your companion's pace or to facilitate praying aloud. After the workout, spend extra time with your companion by sharing a post-workout beverage or snack. If you can't find a willing exercise partner, then take advantage of one who is always with you — your guardian angel. Ask your guardian angel to pray the Rosary with you and listen for your angel's guidance. Reflect on the Glorious Mysteries.

Workout: Complete the **Archangel Level warm-up**. Maintain the warm-up pace (RPE of 2-3), and pray four decades of the Rosary. Transition to the **Archangel Level cool-down** at the beginning of the 5th decade and finish the Rosary. Total workout time should be about 20 minutes, including warm-up and cool-down.

Journal entry: Log your workout in your journal.

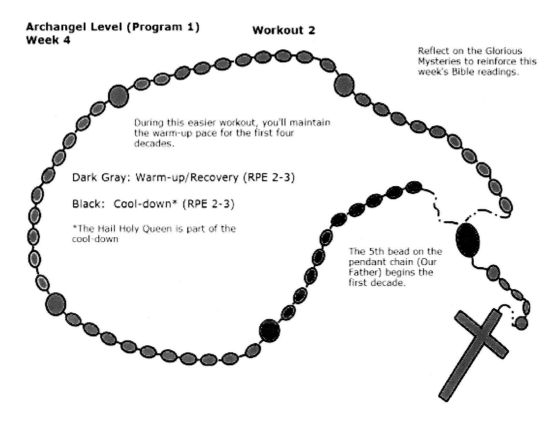

Archangel Level (Program 1)
Week 4

Workout 2

Reflect on the Glorious Mysteries to reinforce this week's Bible readings.

During this easier workout, you'll maintain the warm-up pace for the first four decades.

Dark Gray: Warm-up/Recovery (RPE 2-3)

Black: Cool-down* (RPE 2-3)

*The Hail Holy Queen is part of the cool-down

The 5th bead on the pendant chain (Our Father) begins the first decade.

Workout 3 (5-15 minutes total time):

No structured workout today. Instead, warm-up for 3-5 minutes and spend about 5-10 minutes gently stretching. Pray the Rosary as you stretch, or memorize a verse or two from the Bible that pertains to one of the 20 mysteries.

Journal entry: Log your workout in your journal.

Congratulations! You have completed the Archangel Level (Program 1) of The Rosary Workout™.

Mary's promise: I promise my special protection and the greatest graces to all those who shall recite the Rosary.

Archangel Level (Program 1) Graduation Requirements

Note: You will skip the Archangel Level (Program 2). Your next level is Principality.

You are ready to progress to the Principality Level if you have met the following conditions:

1. You have exercised 3 days each week for 4 continuous weeks.
2. You are able to exercise continuously for 20 minutes but still have energy to go longer. 3. You have little, if any, muscle soreness after your workouts.
4. You have read the Biblical references to each mystery of the Rosary.
5. You are beginning to integrate prayer and exercise by focusing on meditation.
6. If you have not met the conditions above, consider extra study and/or workouts before progressing to the Principality Level. If you have not had time to read the Bible references for each mystery, then set aside some time to do so. If you struggle with the workouts, continue building on the progress you've made so far until you are able to meet the frequency and duration goals above. If you are easily distracted during meditation while exercising, try this: Find a quiet area where you can be by yourself for a few minutes with no distractions. Choose any of the 20 mysteries and pray just one decade of the Rosary. As you pray the 10 Hail Mary's, try to imagine yourself as a bystander, watching the scene of the mystery unfold. Another option is to reflect on a passage from the Bible related to the mystery or to look at a picture or painting depicting the mystery scene. Just pray the one decade and try to focus as much as possible on that mystery. Repeat this exercise a few times each week to help you learn to meditate. Eventually, you'll be able to apply this same focus during your workouts.
7. Reward yourself for reaching your goal.
8. Don't forget to pray to the Choir of Archangels (and any saints to whom you prayed for intercession) to thank them for their assistance in helping you complete this level.

Archangel Level (Program 1) Completion Assignments:

For the Soul: Continue your commitment to monthly Confession. Your assignment this month is to memorize a new prayer. Perhaps this can be a prayer to your patron saint or your guardian angel, a novena prayer, a litany or a prayer for a certain cause that is important to you. You might purchase prayer cards or a prayer book at a Catholic bookstore or parish gift shop. There are also many great online resources.

For the Body: Set a goal to increase your daily activity in some small way every day this month. Park at the back of the parking lot at work, the mall, the grocery store, etc. and walk a little farther. Skip the elevator or escalator and take the stairs. Turn on the stereo or radio and dance around the house for 10 minutes. Take a short walk after a meal to aid digestion. Tackle a chore like washing or waxing your vehicle, trimming the hedges, raking the lawn, washing the outside windows, etc.

Archangel Level (Program 2) Week 1
Increasing duration to 30 minutes with 2 workouts weekly

<u>Note</u> : If you prefer to keep the duration at 20 minutes and increase frequency to three days per week, please go back to **Archangel Level Program 1.**

<u>Spiritual Component</u>: Read the Bible references for each of the **Joyful Mysteries**. (See Appendix C) If you focus on the readings for one mystery a day, the time commitment is just a few minutes each day for five days this week.

Workout 1 (23-24 minutes total time):

Focus: Reflect on the Joyful Mysteries to reinforce this week's Bible readings. Try to establish a consistent rhythm during the main workout to facilitate prayerful meditation.

Today you will add an additional 3-4 minutes to your workout. In past workouts, the transition to the cool-down began with the 5th decade, but today you will continue to pray the 5th decade and the Hail Holy Queen at your base pace._ You may have to make minor adjustments, based on your personal tempo of praying the Rosary.

Workout: After the **Archangel Level warm-up**, increase intensity to your **base pace** (RPE of 3-4). This is a pace which you can comfortably maintain for about 25 minutes. Continue praying the Rosary. When you finish the Rosary, transition to the **Archangel Level cool-down**. During the cool-down period, reflect on the Bible readings for this week and perhaps memorize a verse or two from the readings. The entire workout should take 23-24 minutes, including warm-up and cool-down.

<u>**Journal entry**</u>: Log your workout in your journal.

<u>Note:</u> Refer to this graphic for Weeks 1-3, Workouts 1 and 2

Workout 2 (23-24 minutes total time):

Repeat Workout 1, but do not add additional time today. Total workout time should be 23-24 minutes, including warm-up and cool-down. Try to allow at least one day of rest between workouts.

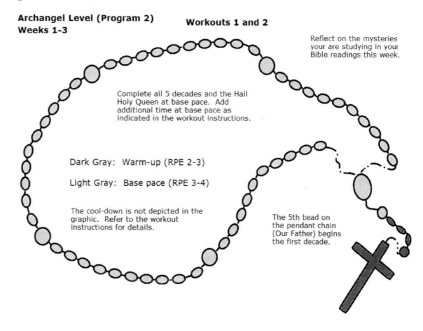

Archangel Level (Program 2) Weeks 1-3

Workouts 1 and 2

Reflect on the mysteries your are studying in your Bible readings this week.

Complete all 5 decades and the Hail Holy Queen at base pace. Add additional time at base pace as indicated in the workout instructions.

Dark Gray: Warm-up (RPE 2-3)

Light Gray: Base pace (RPE 3-4)

The cool-down is not depicted in the graphic. Refer to the workout instructions for details.

The 5th bead on the pendant chain (Our Father) begins the first decade.

Archangel Level (Program 2) Week 2

<u>Spiritual Component</u>: Read the Bible references for the **Luminous Mysteries** (Refer to Appendix C). If you focus on the readings for one mystery a day, the time commitment is just a few minutes for five days each day this week.

Workout 1 (26-28 minutes total):

<u>Focus:</u> Reflect on the Luminous Mysteries today to reinforce this week's Bible readings. As you exercise, try to create a mental picture of each mystery to aid in meditation.

Today you will add an <u>additional</u> 3-4 minutes to the total time of last week's workouts. This time will be added at base pace after you finish the Rosary, so you'll probably need a watch to track the additional time. Use this extra time and the cool-down period to reflect on the Bible readings for this week and perhaps work on memorizing a verse or two from the readings. Another solution is to pray the Rosary at a slower pace, giving you more time for reflection on the readings. Of course, you can simply get lost in your thoughts or enjoy your surroundings.

<u>Workout:</u> After the **Archangel Level warm-up**, increase intensity to your base pace (RPE of 3-4), and pray the Rosary. Add an additional 3-4 minutes at base pace before transitioning to the **Archangel Level cool-down**. Total workout time should be 26-28 minutes, including warm-up and cool-down.

<u>Journal entry</u>: Log your workout in your journal.

Workout 2 (26-28 minutes total):

Repeat Workout 1, but do not add additional time today.

In addition to receiving the spiritual benefits and blessings of regular Rosary prayer, you're also reducing the risk of many life-threatening diseases such as diabetes, cancer, high blood pressure and heart disease.

Archangel Level (Program 2) Week 3

<u>Spiritual Component</u>: Read the Bible passage for the **Sorrowful Mysteries** (Appendix C).

Workout 1 (30 minutes total time):

<u>Focus:</u> Reflect on the Sorrowful Mysteries today. After establishing a comfortable rhythm at your base pace, concentrate on the scene of each mystery. Imagine yourself as an observer, drawing on details from this week's Bible readings. Today you will add an <u>additional</u> 2-4 minutes at base pace to last week's total time. By the end of the week, you should be able to exercise continuously for 30 minutes. Refer to last week's suggestions on how to use the extra workout time to enhance the spiritual aspect of the workout.

Workout: After the **Archangel Level warm-up**, increase intensity to your base pace (RPE of 3-4), and continue praying the Rosary. Add additional time at base pace so that the total workout time is close to 30 minutes, including warm-up and cool-down. Transition to the **Archangel Level cool-down** during the last 3-4 minutes of the workout.

Journal entry: Log your workout in your journal.

Workout 2 (30 minutes total):

If possible, allow at least one day of rest between workouts.

Repeat Workout 1, and try to exercise for 30 minutes today, including warm-up and cool-down. If you aren't able to continue for 30 minutes, keep building on your current workout level every week until you reach 30 minutes. Don't be discouraged if this takes some time. For motivation, look back over your journal to see how far you've come.

Journal entry: Log your workout in your journal.

Exercise benefit: It builds and maintains healthy muscles, bones, and joints.

Archangel Level (Program 2) Week 4

Spiritual Component: Read the Bible references for the **Glorious Mysteries** (Appendix C).

Workout 1 (20-25 minutes total time):

Focus: Today's workout is shorter and easier than usual. An occasional easy workout provides a physical and mental break. To add variety, try a different mode of exercise or invite a friend or family member to accompany you. If you pray the Rosary, take turns reciting the prayers. The traditional method is for one person to say the first half of each prayer and the other(s) to finish it. You may need to decrease the RPE to allow for your companion's pace or to facilitate praying aloud. After the workout, spend extra time with your companion by sharing a post-workout beverage or snack. If you can't find a willing exercise partner, then take advantage of one who is always with you — your guardian angel. Ask your guardian angel to pray the Rosary with you and listen for your angel's guidance. Reflect on the Glorious Mysteries.

Workout: Complete the **Archangel Level warm-up** and maintain the warm-up pace (RPE of 2-3) as you pray the Rosary. Transition to the **Archangel Level cool-down**. Total workout time should be about 20-25 minutes, including warm-up and cool-down.

Journal entry: Log your workout in your journal.

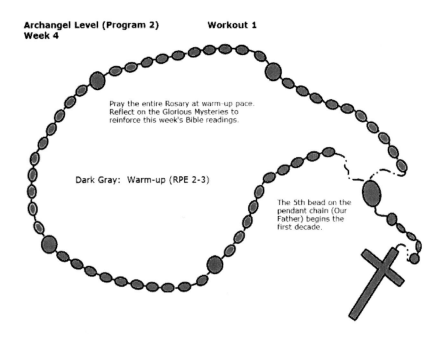

Archangel Level (Program 2)
Week 4

Workout 1

Pray the entire Rosary at warm-up pace.
Reflect on the Glorious Mysteries to
reinforce this week's Bible readings.

Dark Gray: Warm-up (RPE 2-3)

The 5th bead on the
pendant chain (Our
Father) begins the
first decade.

Workout 2 (30 minutes total time):

Focus: Pray the Glorious Mysteries today. Set a comfortable rhythm at your base pace, and concentrate on each mystery. Imagine you are an observer, drawing on details from the Bible readings. After your workout, think of a good deed that you can do for someone today while you spend an extra 5-10 minutes stretching for increased flexibility and relaxation.

Workout: After the **Archangel Level warm-up**, increase intensity to your base pace (RPE of 3-4), and continue praying the Rosary. Add additional time at base pace so that the total workout time is close to 30 minutes, including warm-up and cool-down. Transition to the **Archangel Level cool-down** during the last 3-4 minutes of the workout.

Journal entry: Log your workout in your journal.

Congratulations! You have completed the Archangel Level (Program 2) of The Rosary Workout™.

Mary's promise to those devoted to the Rosary: Whoever shall recite the Rosary devoutly, applying themselves to the consideration of its Sacred Mysteries, shall never be conquered by misfortune. God will not chastise them in His justice, they shall not perish by an unprovided death; if they are just, they shall remain in the grace of God, and become worthy of eternal life.

Archangel Level (Program 2) Graduation Requirements

You are ready to progress to the Principality Level if you have met the following conditions:

1. You have exercised 2 days each week for 4 continuous weeks.
2. You are able to exercise continuously for 30 minutes but still have energy to go longer. 3. You have little, if any, muscle soreness after your workouts.
4. You have read the Biblical references for each mystery of the Rosary.
5. You are beginning to integrate prayer and exercise by focusing on meditation.
6. If you have not met the conditions above, consider extra study and/or workouts before you progress to the Principality Level. If you have not had time to read the Bible references for each mystery, then set aside some time to do so before progressing to the next level. If you struggle with the workouts, continue building on the progress you've made so far until you are able to meet the frequency and duration goals above. If you are easily distracted during meditation while exercising, try this: Find a quiet area where you can be by yourself for a few minutes with no distractions. Choose any of the 20 mysteries and pray just one decade of the Rosary. As you pray the 10 Hail Mary's, try to imagine yourself as a bystander, watching the scene of the mystery unfold. Another suggestion is to reflect on a passage from the Bible related to the mystery or look at a picture or painting depicting the mystery scene. Just pray the one decade and try to focus as much as possible on that mystery. Repeat this exercise a few times each week to help you learn to meditate. Eventually, you'll be able to apply this same focus during your workouts.
7. Reward yourself for reaching your goal.
8. Don't forget to pray to the Choir of Archangels (and any saints to whom you prayed for intercession) to thank them for their assistance in helping you complete this level.

Archangel Level (Program 2) Completion Assignments:

For the Soul: Continue your commitment to monthly Confession. Your assignment this month is to memorize a new prayer. Perhaps this can be a prayer to your patron saint or your guardian angel, a novena prayer, a litany or a prayer for a certain cause that is important to you. You might purchase prayer cards or a prayer book at a Catholic bookstore or parish gift shop. There are also many great online resources.

For the Body: Set a goal to increase your daily activity in some small way every day this month. Park at the back of the parking lot at work, the mall, the grocery store, etc. and walk a little farther. Skip the elevator or escalator and take the stairs. Turn on the stereo or radio and dance around the house for 10 minutes. Take a short walk after a meal to aid digestion. Tackle a chore like washing or waxing your vehicle, trimming the hedges, raking the lawn, washing the outside windows, etc.

Principality Level Workouts:
Third Beginner Level (4 weeks)

Prayer to the **Choir of Principalities:**

By the intercession of St. Michael and the celestial Choir of Principalities may God fill our souls with a true spirit of obedience. Amen.

-From the Chaplet of St. Michael the Archangel

Pray to the Choir of Principalities and your guardian angel for help in completing this level.

Principality Level Summary and Goals:

The Principality Level builds on the foundation of the Angel and Archangel Levels. You are accustomed to regular exercise and Rosary prayer, and you have experienced how their combined rhythms enhance meditation.

I will introduce an exciting exercise principle known as **interval training** during the third week. Interval training in the Principality Level serves three purposes:

1. An increased exercise pace presents a physiological challenge to the body to help it grow stronger.

2. The Rosary prayer marking the interval, the Glory Be (Gloria), lifts the mind to heaven to praise and glorify the Blessed Trinity.

3. The combination of a burst of physical energy with the simultaneous joyful praise to heaven elevates our thoughts and our very being toward God. It is a fitting conclusion after pondering one of the Divine mysteries.

"It is important that the Gloria, the high-point of contemplation, be given due prominence in the Rosary. ...The glorification of the Trinity at the end of each decade, far from being a perfunctory conclusion, takes on its proper contemplative tone, raising the mind as it were to the heights of heaven..." -Pope John Paul II, Apostolic Letter, *Rosary of the Virgin Mary*

A short recovery, or resting period, follows the interval and also serves three purposes:

1. The decreased pace takes the stress off the body, allowing it to return to its previous state.

2. It marks the transition between decades of the Rosary, reminding you that you are about to reflect on a new mystery.

3. It prepares you to resume your base pace and your meditative prayer. Readers of all fitness abilities can benefit from this level as an introduction to interval training and the

corresponding effect on the meditative prayer of the Rosary. Intermediate and advanced exercisers can modify the suggested workout parameters based on their current fitness and may want to begin with the workouts in Week 3.

The Principality Level workouts are designed to merge the two programs of the Archangel Level to reach a common set of goals:

Principality Level Goals:

1. Continue to solidify a habit of regular exercise and meditative Rosary prayer.

2. Increase duration (if you completed Archangel Level Program 1) or frequency (if you completed Archangel Level Program 2) in order to exercise three times weekly for 30 minutes.

3. Introduce interval training as a means to improve fitness and enhance meditative prayer.

Note: If you truly cannot find the time to add a third day of exercise, then you can still complete the level -- simply modify the published workouts to meet your schedule and fitness needs. One option is to increase the duration of the workouts, but don't add more than 5-10 minutes in any given week. No specific workouts are given for this option.

After completing the Principality Level you should be able to:

1. Meditate on the mysteries of the Rosary while exercising 3 times per week

2. Exercise continuously for 30 minutes

3. Complete at least two intervals during a workout

Spiritual Component for the Principality Level:

Beginners in Mary's School of the Rosary: Now that you are familiar with the Bible references for all 20 mysteries, the next step is to view and study artwork depicting each mystery. This engages the part of the brain that processes visual information. In doing so, you follow the example set by St. Louis de Montfort, a great devotee to Mary and the Rosary. He carried a set of banners, each a simple artistic depiction of one of the mysteries. When leading his congregation in Rosary prayer, he displayed the appropriate banner as an aid to meditation.

Obviously an art museum is a good place to look for religious art, but there are many good books and websites on the subject as well. Look for those written from a Catholic perspective to avoid confusion or misinterpretation. It's helpful to study commentaries about religious art depicting the scenes of the mysteries. There are many symbols used in religious paintings and artwork that help deepen your understanding.

The spiritual components for this level are again grouped by the types of mysteries: Joyful,

Luminous, Sorrowful and Glorious. You'll study a different group of mysteries in art form during each of the four weeks of the Principality Level.

<u>Intermediate and advanced students in Mary's School of the Rosary:</u> You may already own several books, holy cards and Scriptural Rosary booklets which depict the mysteries in art. Expand your resources for visual aids to meditation by using some of the ideas listed above.

Exercise Components for the Principality Level:

Frequency: 3 days per week

Duration: 22 – 30 minutes each workout

<u>Note</u>: I make the assumption that you can pray a five-decade Rosary in approximately 18-20 minutes. If it takes you significantly more or less time, modify the workouts to in order to meet the recommended total time.

Intensity:

Warm-up and cool-down: Very Easy to Easy (2-3 on RPE scale)

Base pace: Easy to Moderate (3-4 on the RPE scale)

Interval: Base pace RPE + 1

Recovery: Base pace RPE minus 1

Mode: Any type of rhythmic aerobic exercise (walking, biking, etc.) Use the same mode of exercise that you used in the Angel and Archangel Levels for most of your workouts. If you need variety or a change of pace, feel free to try a different mode of exercise. Limit this to once a week, and keep in mind that a new mode of exercise may require adjustments in RPE and duration.

Principality Level Warm-up: The Principality Level warm-up is the same throughout all the workouts in this level and is therefore listed only once. As you begin the physical portion of the warm-up (RPE of 2-3), you should simultaneously "warm-up" spiritually with a short prayer to the Holy Spirit, your patron saint or the Blessed Mother asking for help in learning to meditate upon each mystery of the Rosary as you exercise. Decide on a Rosary intention based on your own needs or those of others. The warm-up should last about 5 minutes.

<u>Note:</u> You will not pray the Rosary until you finish the warm-up and start the actual workout.

Principality Level Cool-down: The Principality Level cool-down is also the same throughout all the workouts in this level. Slow your pace to an RPE of 2-3 for about 5 minutes. Use this time to reflect on the mysteries, get lost in your thoughts or enjoy your surroundings and the great feeling of accomplishment in finishing your workout.

Stretch: If time allows after your workout, take a few minutes to stretch the major muscle groups you worked during exercise. If you don't have time to stretch, try to fit in a stretching session later in the day or at least 2-3 times each week.

Principality Level Week 1

Spiritual Component: View and study artwork depicting the Joyful Mysteries to aid meditation.

Workout 1 (30 minutes total time):

Focus: Draw on the Bible readings from the Archangel Level and artwork depicting the mysteries to aid in your meditation on the Joyful Mysteries.

Note to those who completed Archangel Level Program 1: From now on, you will add an additional 10 minutes to the 20-minute workouts you did in the last level. The first 5 minutes are a warm-up period. During the next 20 minutes, you'll pray the Rosary while exercising at your base pace. The last 5 minutes is a cool-down period. If a 30-minute workout is too much for you at this point, modify the workout to meet your current abilities. You can also decrease your base pace RPE if this will allow you to meet the 30-minute goal.

Workout: After the **Principality Level Warm-up**, increase intensity to your base pace (RPE of 3-4). This is a pace which you can comfortably maintain for 30 minutes. At the same time, begin the Rosary. After you finish the Rosary (or have exercised for 20 minutes at base pace), transition to the **Principality Level Cool-down**. If you are able to pray the Rosary in fewer than 20 minutes, add additional time at your base pace. The entire workout should take about 30 minutes, including warm-up and cool-down.

Journal entry: Log your workout in your journal.

Note: The graphic on the next page can be applied to all the workouts in Weeks 1-2 of the Principality Level. Modify as needed according to the workout notes. (From now on, the warm-up and cool-down are not part of the graphics)

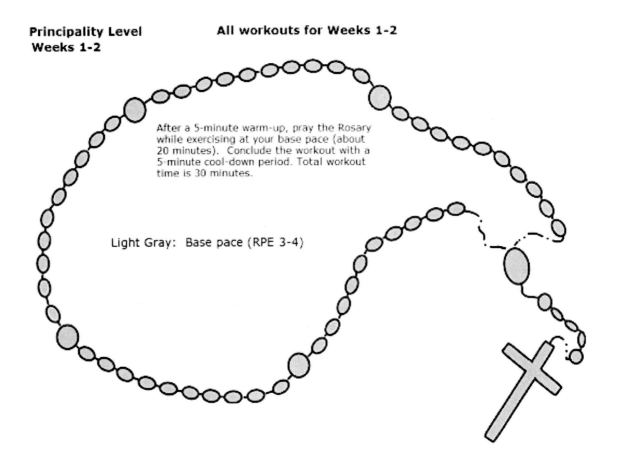

**Principality Level
Weeks 1-2**

All workouts for Weeks 1-2

After a 5-minute warm-up, pray the Rosary while exercising at your base pace (about 20 minutes). Conclude the workout with a 5-minute cool-down period. Total workout time is 30 minutes.

Light Gray: Base pace (RPE 3-4)

Workout 2 (30 minutes total time):

Repeat Workout 1. If possible, allow at least one day of rest between workouts.

Workout 3 (30 minutes total time):

Repeat Workout 1.

<u>Note to those who completed Archangel Level Program 2:</u> This is the first time that you will increase the frequency of your workouts to 3 days per week. Modify the RPE and/or duration as needed to allow your body to adapt to the third weekly workout.

Benefit of devotion to the Rosary: It enriches us with graces and merits.

Benefit of regular exercise: It decreases anxiety and depression and improves psychological well-being.

<u>Spiritual Component</u>: View and study artwork depicting the Luminous Mysteries as an aid to meditation.

Workout 1 (30 minutes total time):

Focus: Use the rhythm of your base pace to clear your mind. Draw on the Bible readings from the Archangel Level and artwork depicting the mysteries to aid in your meditation on the Luminous Mysteries.

Workout: After the **Principality Level Warm-up**, increase intensity to your base pace (RPE of 3-4), and pray the Rosary. After you finish the Rosary (or have exercised for 20 minutes at base pace), transition to the **Principality Level Cool-down**. If you can pray the Rosary in fewer than 20 minutes, add additional time at your base pace. The entire workout should take about 30 minutes, including warm-up and cool-down.

Journal entry: Log your workout in your journal.

Workout 2 (30 minutes total time):

Repeat Workout 1. Try to allow at least one day of rest between workouts.

Workout 3 (30 minutes total time):

Repeat Workout 1.

"Say the Holy Rosary. Blessed be that monotony of Hail Mary's which purifies the monotony of your sins!" -St. Josemaria Escriva

<u>Spiritual Component</u>: View and study artwork depicting the Sorrowful Mysteries as an aid to meditation.

Workout 1 (30 minutes total time):

Focus: This is your first **interval training** workout! The intervals are very short, and you should recover quickly. A graphic of the workout on the next page will help you visualize how the intervals and recovery periods are incorporated with the Rosary prayers. At first it may be a challenge to meditate while remembering what to do next, but the workouts have a definite pattern, and you'll quickly adjust. Draw on the Bible readings from the Archangel Level and artwork depicting the mysteries to aid in your meditation on the Sorrowful

Mysteries. Remember to use your journal to record details of your workout and notes on meditation.

Workout: After the **Principality Level Warm-up**, increase intensity to your base pace (RPE of 3-4) and begin the Rosary. Pray the Apostles' Creed, Our Father, three Hail Mary's, Fatima Prayer and Glory Be. Continue with the 1st mystery announcement, Our Father and 10 Hail Mary's of the first decade.

The first interval starts with the Glory Be at the <u>end of the first decade</u>. As you begin the Glory Be, increase your base pace RPE by one. This is not an all-out effort, but rather a speeding up of your base pace. For instance, if you normally walk, you can jog or power walk (swing your arms and walk like you're late for something important). The goal is to maintain this increased pace through the Glory Be (about 10-15 seconds). Do not rush the prayer in an effort to shorten the interval, but <u>allow the burst of physical energy to intensify your prayer of praise to the Blessed Trinity</u>.

<u>Note:</u> This is a good time to use the **"talk test"** to judge RPE by saying the prayers out loud. If you can only gasp out a few words, you are working too hard. Decrease your effort slightly until you can talk without feeling starved for air.

The next part of the Rosary (Fatima Prayer, 2nd mystery announcement and Our Father) marks your **recovery** period during which you will slow down and catch your breath. Decrease your pace to base pace RPE minus one. (Note that this is actually your interval RPE minus 2.) Try not to stop exercising completely, but do slow down as you continue exercising. As your body recovers, think about the prayers you are saying. You are asking for Jesus' mercy, though the Fatima Prayer, before transitioning to the next decade. The Our Father reminds you of the heavenly origin of the next mystery.

Resume your base pace RPE as you begin the next decade of Hail Mary's. Allow the familiar rhythm of your base pace to clear your mind for meditation.

The second interval begins with the Glory Be <u>at the end of the 3rd decade</u>. Repeat the increased pace as you did with the first interval. Recover during the Fatima Prayer, 4th mystery announcement and Our Father. Resume your base pace during the 4th decade of Hail Mary's. Finish praying the Rosary, then transition to the **Principality Level Cool-down**.

Journal entry: Log your workout in your journal. Include details about the intervals and their effect on your Rosary meditation.

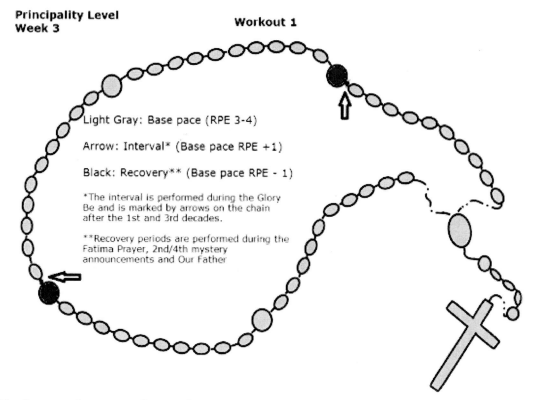

Principality Level Week 3

Workout 1

Light Gray: Base pace (RPE 3-4)

Arrow: Interval* (Base pace RPE +1)

Black: Recovery** (Base pace RPE - 1)

*The interval is performed during the Glory Be and is marked by arrows on the chain after the 1st and 3rd decades.

**Recovery periods are performed during the Fatima Prayer, 2nd/4th mystery announcements and Our Father

Workout 2 (20-30 minutes):

Focus: This workout is intentionally easy to give your body a day of "active rest" and is <u>most effective when done the day after an interval workout</u>. Do not try to exercise at an intensity greater than your base pace RPE minus one. This workout offers an excellent opportunity to practice meditation on the Luminous Mysteries and to devote a few extra minutes to stretching.

Workout: Following the **Principality Level Warm-up**, increase intensity to your recovery pace (base pace RPE minus one) as you pray the Rosary during a 20–30 minute workout (including warm-up and cool-down). For some exercisers, the warm-up pace and the recovery pace are essentially the same. Transition to the **Principality Level Cool-down** during the last five minutes of the workout.

Journal entry: Log your workout in your journal.

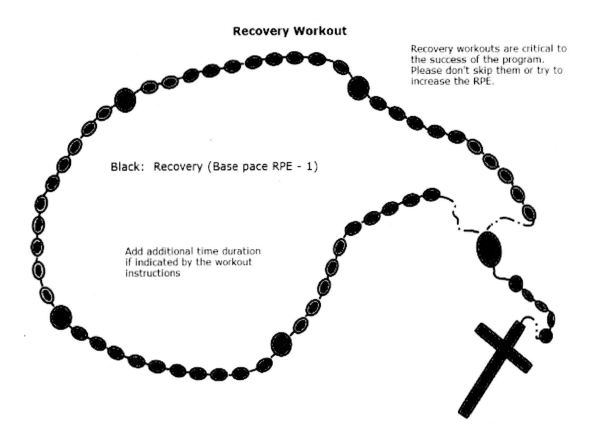

Recovery Workout

Recovery workouts are critical to the success of the program. Please don't skip them or try to increase the RPE.

Black: Recovery (Base pace RPE - 1)

Add additional time duration if indicated by the workout instructions

<u>Note:</u> Refer to this graphic for all Recovery Workouts in this level.

Workout 3 (30 minutes total time):

<u>Focus:</u> Meditate on the Luminous Mysteries as you exercise.

<u>Workout:</u> After the **Principality Level Warm-up**, increase intensity to your base pace (RPE of 3-4), and pray the Rosary. After you finish the Rosary (or have exercised for 20 minutes at base pace), transition to the **Principality Level Cool-down**. If you can pray the Rosary in fewer than 20 minutes, add additional time at your base pace. The entire workout should take about 30 minutes, including warm-up and cool-down. (Find a graphic representation of the this workout in Week 1, Workout 1)

<u>Journal entry</u>: Log your workout in your journal.

Exercise increases self-esteem and self-confidence. It reduces or maintains body weight or body fat, and leads to overall feelings of well-being and good health.

<u>Spiritual Component</u>: View and study artwork depicting the Glorious Mysteries as an aid to meditation.

Workout 1 (30 minutes total time):

Focus: Today's interval workout will add two additional intervals for a total of four. A graphic representation of the workout on the next page will help you visualize how the intervals and recovery periods are incorporated with the Rosary prayers.

Draw on the Bible readings from the Archangel Level and artwork depicting the mysteries to aid in your meditation on the Glorious Mysteries.

Workout: After the **Principality Level Warm-up**, increase intensity to your base pace (RPE of 3-4). At the same time, begin the Rosary. Pray the pendant chain prayers (Apostles' Creed, Our Father, three Hail Mary's, Fatima Prayer and Glory Be). Continue with the 1st mystery announcement, Our Father and 10 Hail Mary's of the first decade.

The first interval starts with the Glory Be at the <u>end of the first decade</u>. As you begin the Glory Be, increase your base pace RPE by one. Recall that this is not an all-out effort, but rather a speeding up of your base pace.

Decrease your pace to base pace RPE minus one and recover during the Fatima Prayer, 2nd mystery announcement and Our Father. Remember to really reflect on the meaning of those prayers as you recover.

Resume your base pace RPE as you begin the 2nd decade of Hail Mary's. Allow the familiar rhythm of your base pace to clear your mind for meditation.

The second, third and fourth intervals repeat the pattern, increasing your pace during the Glory Be <u>at the end of the 2nd, 3rd and 4th decades</u>. Recover during the Fatima Prayer, mystery announcement and Our Father. Resume your base pace and begin meditating on the next mystery during the subsequent decade of Hail Mary's. Finish praying the Rosary, then transition to the **Principality Level Cool-down**.

<u>Journal entry</u>: Log your workout in your journal. Include details about the intervals and their effect on your Rosary meditation.

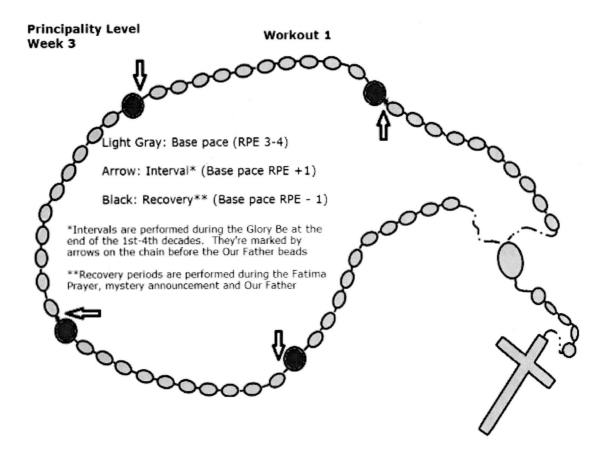

**Principality Level
Week 3**

Workout 1

Light Gray: Base pace (RPE 3-4)

Arrow: Interval* (Base pace RPE +1)

Black: Recovery** (Base pace RPE - 1)

*Intervals are performed during the Glory Be at the end of the 1st-4th decades. They're marked by arrows on the chain before the Our Father beads

**Recovery periods are performed during the Fatima Prayer, mystery announcement and Our Father

Workout 2 (20-30 minutes total time):

Focus: This workout is intentionally easy to give your body a day of "active rest" and is <u>most effective when done the day after an interval workout</u>. Do not try to exercise at an intensity greater than your base pace RPE minus one. Meditate on the Glorious Mysteries, and add an extended stretching session after the cool-down to increase flexibility.

Workout: Following the **Principality Level Warm-up**, increase intensity to your recovery pace (base pace RPE minus one) as you pray the Rosary during a 20–30 minute workout (including warm-up and cool-down). For some exercisers, the warm-up pace and the recovery pace are essentially the same. Transition to the **Principality Level Cool-down** during the last five minutes of the workout.

Journal entry: Log your workout in your journal.

Workout 3 (20-25 minutes total time):

Focus: To add a little variety, try a new mode of exercise for this workout. If you normally walk, dust off your bike and go for a ride. If you usually swim, rent a kayak or try the rowing machine. Limit the total workout time to 20-25 minutes, and adjust the RPE if needed. Meditate on the Glorious Mysteries, and during your cool-down, think of a good deed that you can do for someone today.

Workout: After the **Principality Level Warm-up**, increase RPE to 2-4 and pray the Rosary during a 20-25 minute workout at an easy and enjoyable pace. Transition to the **Principality Level Cool-down** during the last five minutes of the workout.

Journal entry: Log your workout in your journal.

Congratulations! You have completed the Principality Level of The Rosary Workout™. You're ready for the challenging workouts of the Intermediate Series.

Principality Level Graduation Requirements

You are ready to move on to the Intermediate Level if you have met the following conditions:

1. You have exercised 3 days each week for 4 continuous weeks.
2. You are comfortable exercising continuously for 30 minutes.
3. You feel energetic after your workouts, not tired or sore.
4. You can complete at least 2 intervals.
5. You are learning to meditate on the Rosary mysteries during your workouts.
6. If you have not met the conditions above, consider extra study and/or workouts before you progress to the Power Level. If you struggle with the workouts, continue building on the progress you've made so far until you are able to meet the frequency and duration goals above. If you are easily distracted during meditation while exercising, refer to the suggestions in the Archangel Level Graduation Requirements.
7. Reward yourself for reaching your goal.
8. Don't forget to pray to the Choir of Principalities (and any saints to whom you prayed for intercession) to thank them for their assistance in helping you complete this level.

Principality Level Completion Assignments:

For the Soul: Don't forget to go to Confession this month. Learn more about Novenas and pray a Novena for someone who has asked for or needs your prayers. Pamphlets and prayer cards with Novenas are available at Catholic bookstores or search online.

For the Body: Check out these websites for ideas to add variety to your workout routine:
www.acefitness.org/fitfacts
www.fitness.gov

Note: You may not want to progress to the Intermediate Series, and that is perfectly fine. You can still maintain a healthy and beneficial level of fitness. Continue to add challenges to your workouts by occasionally incorporating some of the longer intervals in the Intermediate Series into your routine. Gradually increase the duration of your workouts, if possible, or add an extra day here and there. In any case, do persevere with your exercise routine. You've worked hard to establish this habit — don't let go simply because you can't find extra time to progress through the next levels. Increase your daily activity by parking a distance away from your destination and walking, taking the stairs instead of the elevator, riding your bike instead of driving, etc.

Do realize that you <u>can</u> and <u>should</u> continue to progress in Mary's School of the Rosary. Continue reading, studying and reflecting on the words and examples of Christ in the Bible. Refer to the spiritual component exercises and the end-of-level homework assignments in the Intermediate and Advanced Series for more ideas to improve your spiritual fitness.

Intermediate Series

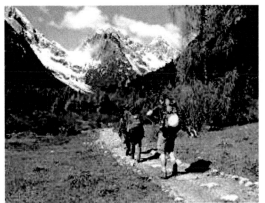

The Intermediate Series builds on the "foundation of rock" laid in the Beginner Series: the integration of exercise and Rosary meditation. Intermediate workouts are exciting because you will use the structure of the Rosary to vary the workouts and vastly improve fitness through interval training. Rosary meditation is enhanced because the intervals increase the focus on each mystery.

There are three levels in the Intermediate Series: **Power**, **Virtue** and **Dominion**. These levels incorporate periodization and are designed to prevent injury, add variety and optimize training adaptation.

To begin the Intermediate Series you should be at an intermediate level in physical fitness and in Mary's School of praying the Rosary. Refer to the definitions of the **Intermediate exerciser** and the **Intermediate Level of Mary's School**, if needed.

If you exercise regularly and want to skip the Beginner workouts, consider that praying the Rosary and meditating while you exercise is a skill that must be practiced and doesn't come naturally. I highly recommend that you modify your current workout routine to include two or three Beginner workouts each week. Increase the duration and suggested RPE as needed, and follow the spiritual exercises until you are comfortable with Rosary meditation during steady-state exercise. This may not take the full 12 weeks that the Beginner series requires.

The Intermediate Series is probably the most difficult level to master. Beginners are usually eager and motivated, but intermediates may need encouragement to continue the program, especially when trying to fit workouts and spiritual assignments into busy lives.

Jesus addresses these difficulties in the Parable of the Sower:

"The seed sown among thorns is the one who hears the Word, then worldly anxieties and the lure of riches choke the Word and it bears no fruit." (Matthew 13: 22)

To overcome such difficulties, The Rosary Workout™ prioritizes care of the body and soul through the periodized workouts and defined spiritual goals of the Intermediate Series. You'll find encouragement in the physical fitness gains from interval training. Likewise, progressing to the Intermediate Level of Mary's School of the Rosary will expand your understanding of the mysteries. Now that you've mastered the basics of Rosary prayer and meditation, the focus will shift to the Word of God in the Bible. The spiritual component of the Intermediate Series includes a 12-week study of the Gospels. Since there are four Gospels, you will focus on one Gospel for three weeks.

If you have already studied the Gospels, feel free to modify the spiritual goals. An in-depth study of the Old Testament, the Book of Psalms, the Epistles, or Revelation will certainly provide inspiration for meditative prayer.

Bible Translations and Study Guides:

It's important that the Bible you use for study is a Catholic Bible. Protestant versions delete several books and change the wording in a few passages. There are several different translations of the Catholic Bible, and the version used is a matter of personal preference. There is an excellent article on Bible Versions and Commentaries at:
www.ewtn.com/expert/answers/bible_versions.htm

If you don't own a Bible or want to view a different version, you can find it online:
New American Catholic Bible: **www.usccb.org/nab/bible**
Douay-Rheims Catholic Bible: **www.drbo.org**
Revised Standard Version (RSV) Catholic Edition:
www.ewtn.com/devotionals/biblesearch.asp

To guide your study of the Bible during this and future levels, it's helpful to join a Bible study group if your parish offers one. If you can't join a group, there are other ways to study the Bible at home. Search the internet for online Catholic Bible studies, or ask your parish priest or RCIA coordinator for recommendations. You might purchase or borrow a Catholic Study Bible which includes the books of the Bible plus extensive commentary. The most popular are the *Navarre Bible*, the *Ignatius Study Bible* and the *Douay-Rheims Haydock Study Bible*.

Note: From now on, you'll pray the Rosary at least three times a week during your workouts. This makes you eligible to join the Confraternity of the Holy Rosary, whose members pledge to pray all 15 traditional mysteries each week. (The addition of the Luminous mysteries is encouraged, but not required.) This organization can be traced back to St. Dominic, the great Rosary saint. There are many powerful promises, benefits and indulgences for members of this confraternity, and there's no cost to join. Learn more at their website:
www.rosary-center.org

Power Level Workouts:
First Intermediate Level (4 weeks)

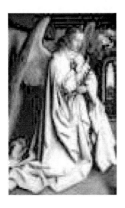

Prayer to the **Choir of Powers:**

By the intercession of St. Michael and the celestial Choir of Powers may the Lord protect our souls against the snares and temptations of the devil. Amen.

-From the Chaplet of St. Michael the Archangel

Pray to the Choir of Powers and your own Guardian angel to ask their assistance in completing this level.

Power Level Summary and Goals:

Up until now your workouts have been focused on habit formation and learning to pray and meditate on the Rosary while exercising. You have also practiced interval training. Now you're ready to add POWER by increasing the duration and frequency of intervals. Each interval begins with the Glory Be (Gloria), which is a most appropriate prayer for a burst of energy, as you discovered in the Principality Level.

Power Level Goals:

1. Progress to a more challenging level of exercise by increasing the duration and frequency of intervals (bursts of increased intensity).

2. Incorporate periodization in this four-week micro-cycle, building to a peak at Week 3, followed by a recovery week.

3. Apply the concept of recovery to interval training and weekly workouts.

4. Learn to use the structure of the Rosary to mark interval and recovery sets while maintaining prayerful meditation.

5. Begin an in-depth study of the four gospels

After completing the Power Level you should be able to:

1. Pray the Rosary while exercising for 30 minutes, 3 days each week

2. Complete 3-5 intervals during an interval workout (at least 20-30 seconds each)

3. Attain a deeper understanding of the four gospels

Spiritual Component for the Power Level:

You'll spend the first three weeks studying the gospel of Matthew, before progressing to the Gospel of Mark in the 4th week. Refer to the section on **Bible Translations and Study Guides**, if needed.

Exercise Components for the Power Level:

Frequency: 3 days per week

Duration: 20-30 minutes each workout

Note 1: All total workout times include warm-up and cool-down

Note 2: I make the assumption that you can pray a five-decade Rosary in approximately 18-20 minutes. If needed, modify the workouts to accommodate your personal tempo.

Intensity:

Warm-up and Cool-down: Easy to Moderate (3-4 on RPE scale)

Base pace: Moderate to Somewhat Hard (4-5 on RPE scale)

Interval: Base pace RPE + 1

Recovery: Base pace RPE minus 1

Mode: Any type of rhythmic aerobic exercise (walking, biking, etc.) Use the same mode of exercise that you used in the Beginner Levels for most of your workouts. If you need variety or a change of pace, feel free to try a different mode of exercise. Just keep in mind that a new mode of exercise may affect your RPE or workout duration.

Power Level Warm-up: The Power Level warm-up is the same throughout all the workouts in this level and is therefore listed only once. As you begin the physical portion of the warm-up, you should also "warm-up" spiritually. Begin exercise at an RPE of 3-4 (this is an increase from the Beginner Level warm-up RPE) while you say a short prayer to the Holy Spirit, your patron saint or the Blessed Mother asking for help in learning to meditate upon each mystery of the Rosary as you exercise. Decide on a Rosary intention based on your own needs or those of others. The warm-up should last at least 5 minutes to prepare you for the higher-intensity intermediate workouts.

Note: You will not begin praying the Rosary until you finish the warm-up and start the actual workout.

Power Level Cool-down: The Power Level cool-down is also the same throughout all the workouts in this level. Slow your pace to an RPE of 3-4 (also an increase from the Beginner Level cool-down RPE) for 3-5 minutes. Use this time to reflect on the mysteries, think of a good deed you can do today, or enjoy your surroundings and the great feeling of accomplishment in finishing your workout.

Stretch: If time allows after your workout, take a few minutes to stretch the major muscle groups you worked during exercise. If you don't have time to stretch, try to fit in a stretching session later in the day or at least 2-3 times each week. For more information, refer to the section on stretching

Power Level Week 1

Spiritual Component: This week you will begin your study of the Gospel of Matthew. Refer to the section on **Bible Translations and Study Guides**, if needed. If you study a chapter or two a day, you'll easily finish in three weeks. Take more time if you need it as this is an important tool for Rosary meditation and should not be rushed.

Workout 1 - Intervals (30 minutes total time):

Focus: This interval workout builds on those you accomplished in the Principality Level. The duration of the intervals is increased to include all the prayers marked by the isolated bead between decades: The Glory Be, Fatima Prayer, mystery announcement and Our Father. As you increase your exercise pace during the interval, allow the corresponding prayers to lift your thoughts to heaven as you praise and glorify the Trinity, ask for God's mercy and transition to the next mystery. During the recovery, return your focus to meditation on the new mystery.

A graphic representation following the workout description will help you visualize how the intervals and recovery periods are incorporated with the Rosary prayers. At first it may be a challenge to meditate while remembering what to do next, but the workouts have a definite pattern, and you'll quickly adjust.

Note: Warm-up and cool-down periods are no longer depicted on the graphics

Workout: After the **Power Level Warm-up**, increase intensity to base pace (RPE of 4-5). This is a pace which you can comfortably maintain for 30 minutes. At the same time, begin the Rosary. Pray the Apostles' Creed, Our Father, three Hail Mary's, Fatima Prayer and Glory Be. Continue with the 1st mystery announcement, Our Father and 10 Hail Mary's of the first decade.

The first interval starts with the Glory Be <u>at the end of the first decade</u>. As you begin the Glory Be, increase your base pace RPE by one. This is not an all-out effort, but rather a speeding up of your base pace. For instance, if you normally walk, you can jog or power walk (swing your arms and walk like you're late for something important). The goal is to maintain this increased pace through the Glory Be, Fatima Prayer, 2nd mystery announcement and Our Father (about 30-60 seconds). Do not rush the prayers in an effort to shorten the interval. This is a good time to use the "talk test" to judge RPE by saying the prayers out loud. If you are able to just gasp out a few words, you are working too hard.

Decrease your effort slightly until you can talk without feeling as if you are starved for air. Modify the interval duration if needed. The ten Hail Mary's of the 2nd decade mark the recovery period as you slow down and catch your breath. Do not stop exercising; rather, decrease your pace to base pace RPE minus one. (Note that this is actually your interval RPE minus 2.) As you relax and recover, meditate on the new mystery.

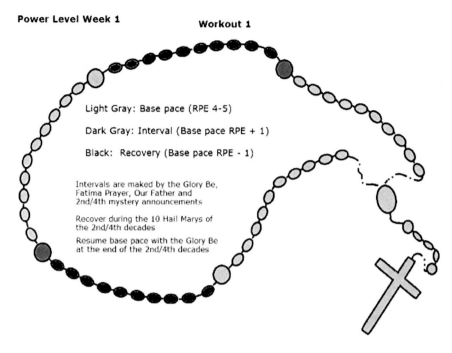

Power Level Week 1 — **Workout 1**

Light Gray: Base pace (RPE 4-5)

Dark Gray: Interval (Base pace RPE + 1)

Black: Recovery (Base pace RPE - 1)

Intervals are marked by the Glory Be, Fatima Prayer, Our Father and 2nd/4th mystery announcements

Recover during the 10 Hail Marys of the 2nd/4th decades

Resume base pace with the Glory Be at the end of the 2nd/4th decades

Resume your base pace RPE with the Glory Be <u>at the end of the second decade</u>. Take more time to recover if needed. Continue base pace through the 10 Hail Mary's of the third decade.

The second interval will begin with the Glory Be <u>at the end of the third decade</u>. Repeat the increased pace as you did with the first interval. The ten Hail Mary's of the fourth decade mark your recovery period and meditation on the fourth mystery.

Resume your base pace RPE with the Glory Be <u>at the end of the fourth decade</u>. Finish praying the Rosary at base pace, then transition to the **Power Level Cool-down**.

<u>**Journal entry**</u>: Log your workout in your journal. Since you're using the Rosary prayers as a timing method for intervals and recovery time, use them as references in your journal. Include details about the intervals — at what point did you became tired during the interval? How long did it last? When were you able to resume your base pace? When did you feel like you were ready for another interval? Add notes about revelations or thoughts you experienced during your Rosary meditation.

Workout 2 – Recovery (20-30 minutes total time):

Focus: This workout is designed to be easy and serves as an active recovery following your high-intensity interval workout. <u>It's most effective when done the day after an interval workout.</u> Remember that adaptation occurs during recovery and not during the overload (interval workouts). Do not skip these recovery workouts or try to exercise at an intensity greater than your base pace RPE minus one. Recovery workouts offer an excellent opportunity to practice meditation on the mysteries.

Workout: After the **Power Level Warm-up**, increase intensity to recovery pace (base pace RPE minus one) as you pray the Rosary during a 20–30 minute workout (including warm-up and cool-down). For some exercisers, the warm-up pace and recovery pace are essentially the same. Transition to the **Power Level Cool-down** during the last 5 minutes of the workout.

Journal entry: Log your workout in your journal

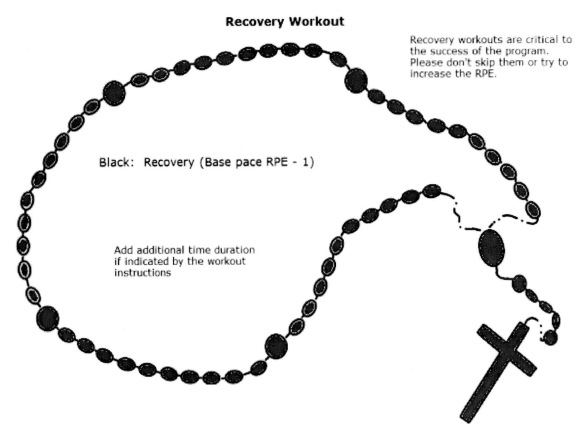

Recovery Workout

Recovery workouts are critical to the success of the program. Please don't skip them or try to increase the RPE.

Black: Recovery (Base pace RPE - 1)

Add additional time duration if indicated by the workout instructions

Note: Refer to this graphic for all recovery workouts in the Intermediate Series.

Workout 3 – Base Pace Training (30 minutes total time):

Focus: Base pace training workouts will follow recovery workouts in the Power Level. The goal is to maintain your base pace as you pray the Rosary and focus on meditation. Use the steady rhythm of your constant pace and the repeated Hail Mary's to clear your mind and enhance the focus on each mystery.

Workout: After completing the **Power Level Warm-up**, increase intensity to your base pace (RPE of 4-5), and pray the Rosary during a 30-minute workout (including warm-up and cool-down). Transition to the **Power Level Cool-down** during the last 5 minutes of the workout

Journal entry: Log your workout in your journal

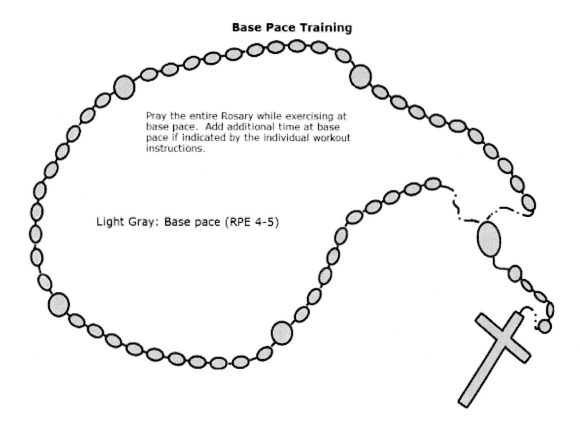

Base Pace Training

Pray the entire Rosary while exercising at base pace. Add additional time at base pace if indicated by the individual workout instructions.

Light Gray: Base pace (RPE 4-5)

Note: Refer to this graphic for all base pace training workouts in the Intermediate Series

"The Rosary is a powerful weapon to put the demons to flight and to keep oneself from sin... If you desire peace in your hearts, in your homes, and in your country, assemble each evening to recite the Rosary. Let not even one day pass without saying it, no matter how burdened you may be with cares and labors." -Pope Pius XI, *The Increasing Evils, Encyclical on the Rosary*

<u>Spiritual Component:</u> Continue your study of the Gospel of Matthew.

Workout 1 – Intervals (30 minutes total time):

<u>**Focus:**</u> This is your second interval workout, and the goal is to complete three intervals. Refer to your journal entry for Workout 1, Week 1 if needed.

<u>**Workout:**</u> After completing the **Power Level Warm-up**, increase intensity to your base pace (RPE of 4-5) and begin praying the Rosary.

The first interval starts with the Glory Be at the end of the <u>first</u> decade. Increase your base pace **RPE** by one and maintain this increased pace through the Glory Be, Fatima Prayer, 2nd mystery announcement and Our Father (about 30-60 seconds).

Recover during the 10 Hail Mary's of the 2nd decade by decreasing the intensity to base pace RPE minus one as you meditate on the 2nd mystery.

The second interval begins with the Glory Be at the end of the 2nd decade. Repeat the increased pace as you did with the first interval. The 3rd decade of 10 Hail Mary's marks the recovery period.

The third interval begins with the Glory Be at the end of the 3rd decade. Repeat the increased pace as you did with the first two intervals. The rest of the 4th decade (10 Hail Mary's) marks the recovery period.

Resume your base pace RPE with the Glory Be <u>at the end of the 4th decade</u>. Transition to the **Power Level Cool-down** after you finish praying the Rosary.

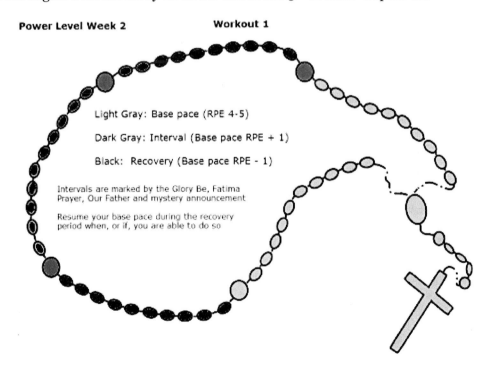

Power Level Week 2   **Workout 1**

Light Gray: Base pace (RPE 4-5)

Dark Gray: Interval (Base pace RPE + 1)

Black: Recovery (Base pace RPE - 1)

Intervals are marked by the Glory Be, Fatima Prayer, Our Father and mystery announcement

Resume your base pace during the recovery period when, or if, you are able to do so

<u>Note1</u>: You can skip or shorten any interval if needed.

<u>Note 2</u>: If you recover quickly and don't need to use the entire decade as a recovery period, feel free to resume your base pace when you're ready to do so.

<u>**Journal entry**</u>: Log your workout in your journal.

Workout 2 – Recovery (20-30 minutes total time):

<u>**Focus:**</u> This easy workout is most effective when done the day after an interval workout. Reflect on what you've learned in your Bible study as you meditate.

<u>**Workout:**</u> After completing the **Power Level Warm-up**, increase intensity to your recovery pace (base pace RPE minus one) and pray the Rosary during a 20–30 minute workout. Transition to the **Power Level Cool-down** in the last 5 minutes.

<u>**Journal entry**</u>: Log your workout in your journal.

Workout 3 – Base Pace Training (30 minutes total time):

<u>**Focus:**</u> Use the steady rhythm of your constant pace and the repeated Hail Mary's to clear your mind and enhance the focus on each mystery.

<u>**Workout:**</u> After completing the **Power Level Warm-up**, increase intensity to your base pace (RPE of 4-5), and pray the Rosary during a 30-minute workout. Transition to the **Power Level Cool-down** in the last 5 minutes of the workout.

<u>**Journal entry**</u>: Log your workout in your journal.

Mary's Promise: All who recite the Rosary are my children, and brothers and sisters of my only Son, Jesus Christ.

Power Level Week 3 (Peak Week)

This week is the "peak week" in the 4-week microcycle (see the section on **Periodization** for more information). You have slowly increased the amount of training over the past two weeks, and this week will be the most challenging in this level.

<u>Spiritual Component</u>: If you've been studying a chapter or two a day, you should finish the Gospel of Matthew by the end of this week. Take more time if you need it as this is an important tool for Rosary meditation and should not be rushed.

Workout 1 – Intervals (30 minutes total time):

<u>**Focus:**</u> Today you'll increase the number of intervals to four. Take advantage of the recovery

periods to focus on meditation.

Workout: After completing the **Power Level Warm-up**, increase intensity to your base pace (RPE of 4-5) and begin praying the Rosary.

The first interval starts with the Glory Be at the end of the <u>first</u> decade. Increase your base pace RPE by one and maintain this increased pace through the Glory Be, Fatima Prayer, 2nd mystery announcement and Our Father (about 30-60 seconds).

Recover during the 10 Hail Mary's of the 2nd decade by decreasing the intensity to base pace RPE minus one as you meditate on the 2nd mystery.

Repeat this pattern at the end of the 2nd, 3rd, and 4th decades. The rest of the Rosary marks your recovery period. Transition to the **Power Level Cool-down** at the end of the Rosary.

Note1: Skip or shorten any interval if needed.

Note 2: If you recover quickly and don't need to use the entire decade as a recovery period, feel free to resume your base pace when you're ready to do so.

Journal entry: Log your workout in your journal. Include details about the intervals—at what point did you became tired during the interval? How long did it last? When were you able to resume your base pace? When did you feel like you were ready for another interval? Be sure to add notes about any revelations or thoughts you experienced during your Rosary meditation.

Power Level Week 3   **Workout 1**

Light Gray: Base pace (RPE 4-5)

Dark Gray: Interval (Base pace RPE + 1)

Black: Recovery (Base pace RPE - 1)

Intervals are marked by the Glory Be, Fatima Prayer, Our Father and mystery announcement

Resume your base pace during the recovery period when, or if, you are able to do so

Workout 2 – Recovery (20-30 min. total time):

Focus: This easy workout is most effective when done the day after an interval workout. Reflect on what you've learned in your Bible study as you meditate.

Workout: After completing the **Power Level Warm-up**, increase intensity to your recovery pace (base pace RPE minus one) as you pray the Rosary during a 20–30 minute workout. Transition to the **Power Level Cool-down** during the last 5 minutes.

Journal entry: Log your workout in your journal.

Workout 3 - Intervals (30 minutes):

Focus: Today's workout will consist of five intervals. This is your second interval workout this week since it's a peak week. If you're not feeling up to two interval workouts in one week, complete as many intervals as you can, then transition to base pace for the rest of the workout.

By now you should be accustomed to the pattern of intervals and recovery periods. This new rhythm creates a natural transition between decades to the meditation period of ten Hail Mary's that follows.

Workout: After the **Power Level Warm-up**, increase intensity to your base pace (RPE of 4-5) and begin the Rosary. Pray the Apostles' Creed, Our Father and three Hail Mary's.

The **first interval** is different today. It starts with the Glory Be <u>after the three Hail Mary's of the pendant chain</u>. Maintain the increased pace through the end of the Our Father (30-60 seconds).

The 10 Hail Mary's of the <u>first decade</u> mark your recovery period. Decrease your pace to base pace RPE minus one.

The remaining four intervals begin with the Glory Be at the end of the 1st, 2nd, 3rd, and 4th decades. Repeat the increased pace as you did with the first interval. The 10 Hail Mary's following each interval are the recovery periods. Finish with the Hail Holy Queen and transition to the **Power Level Cool-down**.

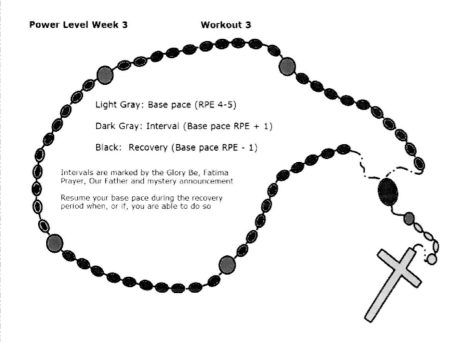

Power Level Week 3   Workout 3

Light Gray: Base pace (RPE 4-5)

Dark Gray: Interval (Base pace RPE + 1)

Black: Recovery (Base pace RPE - 1)

Intervals are marked by the Glory Be, Fatima Prayer, Our Father and mystery announcement

Resume your base pace during the recovery period when, or if, you are able to do so

Journal entry: Log your workout in your journal.

"Lack of activity destroys the good condition of every human being, while movement and methodical physical exercise save it and preserve it." - Plato

Power Level Week 4 (Recovery Week)

This is a "recovery week" in the 4-week microcycle of the Power Level. Workouts are easier and include a few changes for variety. This periodization model (increasing intensity for 3 weeks, followed by a recovery week) will be used for the rest of the workouts in the program.

Spiritual Component: Begin your study of the Gospel of Mark this week.

Workout 1 - Recovery (20-30 minutes total time):

Focus: During the cool-down, think of a good deed you can perform today.

Workout: After completing the **Power Level Warm-up**, increase intensity to your recovery pace (base pace RPE minus one) as you pray the Rosary during a 20–30 minute workout. Transition to the **Power Level Cool-down** during the last 5 minutes.

Journal entry: Log your workout in your journal.

Workout 2 – Base Pace Training (30 minutes total time):

Focus: Try a different mode of exercise to keep things fresh. During the cool-down, pray for someone you dislike or avoid.

Workout: After the **Power Level Warm-up**, attain base pace (RPE of 4-5), and pray the Rosary during a 30-minute workout. Transition to the **Power Level Cool-down** during the last 5 minutes.

Journal entry: Log your workout in your journal.

Workout 3 - Recovery (20-30 minutes total time):

Focus: Easy workout today, so invite a friend or family member to accompany you. If you can't find a willing exercise partner, ask your guardian angel to pray the Rosary with you.

Workout: After completing the **Power Level Warm-up**, increase intensity to your recovery pace (base pace RPE minus one) as you pray the Rosary during a 20–30 minute workout. Transition to the **Power Level Cool-down** during the last 5 minutes.

Journal entry: Log your workout in your journal.

Congratulations! You have conquered the Power Level of The Rosary Workout™. You're burning more calories during each workout, improving speed and increasing overall fitness. You're also using two of the body's fuel sources: stored fat and glycogen (carbohydrates stored in the muscles and liver.)

Power Level Graduation Requirements

You are ready to move on to the Virtue Level if you have met the following conditions:

1. You have exercised 3 days each week for 4 continuous weeks.
2. You are able to complete 3-5 intervals.
3. You have no symptoms of overtraining.
4. You have begun to study the four gospels.
5. If you have not met the conditions above, consider extra study and/or workouts before moving to the Virtue Level. Perhaps an extra week of short, easy workouts will restore your motivation. If you have not started an in-depth study of the gospels, then mark a date on your calendar to begin. It may take several months to study all four gospels, and that's fine. The important thing is to set aside some time a few days each week to devote to Bible study.
6. Reward yourself for reaching your goal.
7. Pray to the Choir of Powers to thank them for their assistance in completing this level.

Power Level Completion Assignments:

<u>For the Soul:</u> Continue your monthly commitment to the Sacrament of Confession. Learn more about the Stations of the Cross, and visit a Catholic church to pray the stations (on Friday if possible). Call ahead to ensure the church will be open. During Lent, many parishes pray the Stations of the Cross publicly as a group, but anyone can pray the stations privately. The stations are usually depicted on the walls around the church. Bring a prayer book on the Stations to help guide your prayer and meditation or print an online guide.

<u>For the Body:</u> If you usually drink more than one cup of coffee a day, try to substitute hot tea occasionally. Tea provides an energy boost and is loaded with disease-fighting antioxidants.

If you drink more than 8 oz. of soda a day (one mini can or half a regular can), try cutting back gradually. Soda contains excessive amounts of sugar that can result in rapid increases or decreases in blood sugar levels that may lower your energy and motivation to work out. The calories from soda are considered "empty" calories. Even diet soda can cause health problems when consumed in excess. Instead, drink water when you're thirsty. Add a wedge of lemon, lime, orange or fresh/frozen berries to flavor the water if you don't like it plain.

Virtue Level Workouts: Second Intermediate Level (4 weeks)

Prayer to the **Choir of Virtues:**

By the intercession of St. Michael and the celestial Choir of Virtues may the Lord preserve us from evil and falling into temptation. Amen.

-From the Chaplet of St. Michael the Archangel

Pray to the Choir of Virtues and your guardian angel for assistance in completing this level.

Virtue Level Summary and Goals:

The Virtue Level adds an extra workout for a frequency of four days per week. Interval workouts increase in both frequency and duration. Your study of the four Gospels continues.

Unstructured Time:

From now on, the workouts will include Rosary prayer three times each week. The fourth weekly workout adds an option for a new concept I'm introducing in this level: **unstructured time**. This is an alternative to praying the Rosary during exercise. Of course, you can pray the Rosary during all your workouts if you prefer. The unstructured time concept simply provides a break from the focused meditation that you've been practicing. It's also an opportunity to watch TV, listen to music or just let your thoughts wander during a workout. Here are a few ideas for unstructured time:

- Memorize a new prayer or Bible verse
- Learn a different type of prayer that uses the Rosary, like the Divine Mercy Chaplet
- Spend a few minutes meditating on just one mystery of the Rosary, perhaps one that you usually can't visualize
- Relax and simply put yourself in God's presence; listen for His voice (this is a good practice for recovery workouts)
- Exercise with a friend or family member
- Listen to your favorite music
- Plan a healthy meal or snack
- Simply get lost in your thoughts or enjoy your surroundings
- Use a heart rate monitor and track your heart rate during exercise
- Try contemplative prayer:

"Contemplative prayer seeks Him 'whom my soul loves'. It is Jesus, and in Him, the Father. We seek Him, because to desire Him is always the beginning of love, and we seek Him in that pure faith which causes us to be born of Him and to live in Him. In this inner prayer we can still meditate, but our attention is fixed on the Lord Himself." (CCC Section 2709)

Contemplative prayer is not easily mastered, so seek advice from a trusted spiritual advisor or find inspiration through contemplative saints. Visit a Catholic bookstores or search online.

Virtue Level Goals:

1. Increase frequency to 4 days per week.

Note: If you cannot exercise four times a week, you can still complete the Virtue Level. Accomplish the workouts in order, but only do three workouts each week. The 4th workout for Week 1 will become the 1st workout for Week 2, etc. Obviously, this will take more than 4 weeks, and the peak and recovery weeks won't line up. Modify the program as needed to fit your schedule. If possible, increase the duration of the Virtue Level workouts by adding 5 minutes to the workouts each week until you reach a total workout time of 50 minutes. Frequent journal entries will help you plan the workouts. <u>Specific instructions are not included for these modifications.</u>

2. Increase the intensity and duration of intervals.

3. Continue your in-depth study of the four gospels

After completing the Virtue Level you should be able to:

1. Pray the Rosary during exercise for 30 minutes, 4 days each week.

2. Increase interval pace to base pace RPE + 2

3. Attain a deeper understanding of the four Gospels.

Spiritual Component for the Virtue Level:

You'll spend the first two weeks continuing your study of the Gospel of Mark, before progressing to the Gospel of Luke on the 3rd week. Refer to the section on **Bible Translations and Study Guides**, if needed.

Exercise Components for the Virtue Level:

Frequency: Increase to 4 days per week

Duration: 30 minutes per workout

<u>Note 1</u>: All total workout times include warm-up and cool-down

<u>Note 2</u>: I make the assumption that you can pray a five-decade Rosary in approximately 18-20 minutes. Modify the workouts if needed to accommodate your personal tempo.

Intensity:

Warm-up and Cool-down: Easy to Moderate (3-4 on RPE scale)

Base pace: Moderate to Somewhat Hard (4-5 on RPE scale)

Interval: Base pace RPE + 2

Recovery: Base pace RPE minus 1

<u>Note</u>: Experienced exercisers may adjust the RPE suggestions above

Mode: Any type of rhythmic aerobic exercise. Try different modes of exercise to add variety and improve fitness.

Virtue Level Warm-up: The Virtue Level warm-up is the same throughout all the workouts in this level and is therefore listed only once. During the physical portion of the warm-up, you should also "warm-up" spiritually. Begin exercise at an RPE of 3-4 while you say a short prayer to the Holy Spirit, your patron saint or the Blessed Mother asking for help in meeting your physical and spiritual goals. Decide on a Rosary intention based on your own needs or those of others. The warm-up should last at least 5 minutes. You are ready to begin your workout with the opening prayer of the Rosary, The Apostles' Creed.

Virtue Level Cool-down: The Virtue Level cool-down is also the same throughout all the workouts in this level. Slow your pace to an RPE of 3-4 for about 5 minutes. Use this time to reflect on the mysteries, think of a good deed you can do today, or enjoy your surroundings and the great feeling of accomplishment in finishing your workout.

Stretch: If time allows after your workout, take a few minutes to stretch the major muscle groups you worked during exercise. If you don't have time to stretch, try to fit in a stretching session later in the day or at least 2-3 times each week.

Virtue Level Week 1

Spiritual Component: Continue your study of the Gospel of Mark.

Workout 1 - Intervals (30 minutes total time):

Focus: This workout consists of five intervals. Recall that an interval includes the Glory Be, Fatima Prayer, mystery announcement and Our Father. (Refer to your journal entry for Week 3, Workout 3 in the Power Level if needed.)   If you skipped or shortened the intervals during your last workout, modify the interval workouts in the Virtue Level until you can complete all five at base pace RPE + 1.

If you are able to complete all five intervals at base pace RPE + 1, you're ready to tackle the Virtue Level goal: increasing interval pace to base pace RPE + 2. Use the "talk test" to judge RPE by saying the prayers out loud. You may need to shorten the duration of the interval or return to your "old" interval pace (base pace RPE + 1) for subsequent intervals.

During the interval, allow the corresponding prayers to lift your thoughts to heaven as you praise and glorify the Trinity, ask for God's mercy and transition to the next mystery. As you recover, return your focus to meditation on the new mystery. Your increasing understanding of the Bible through guided study will enhance meditation.

Workout: After the **Virtue Level Warm-up**, increase intensity to your base pace (RPE of 4-5) and begin the Rosary. Pray the Apostles' Creed, Our Father and three Hail Mary's.

The **first interval** starts with the Glory Be after the three Hail Mary's of the pendant chain. Interval pace is base pace RPE + 2. The 10 Hail Mary's of the 1st decade mark your recovery period. Decrease your pace to base pace RPE minus one. If you recover before the end of the decade, resume your base pace.

The next four intervals begin with the Glory Be at the end of the 1st, 2nd 3rd and 4th decades and end with the Our Father. The 10 Hail Mary's following each interval are the recovery periods. Finish with the Hail Holy Queen and transition to the **Virtue Level Cool-down**.

Journal entry: Log your workout in your journal.

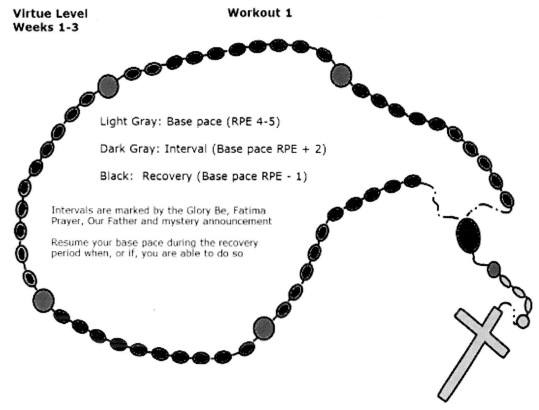

**Virtue Level
Weeks 1-3**

Workout 1

Light Gray: Base pace (RPE 4-5)

Dark Gray: Interval (Base pace RPE + 2)

Black: Recovery (Base pace RPE - 1)

Intervals are marked by the Glory Be, Fatima Prayer, Our Father and mystery announcement

Resume your base pace during the recovery period when, or if, you are able to do so

Workout 2 – Recovery (30 minutes total time):

Focus: This workout is designed to be easy and serves as an active recovery following your high-intensity interval workout. It's most effective when done the day after an interval workout. Recovery workouts are a very important part of a periodized training program because adaptation occurs during recovery and not during the overload (interval workouts). Do not skip these workouts or increase the suggested RPE.

Note: There are no graphics for recovery workouts in the Virtue Level. Refer to the recovery workout graphic in the Power Level, or simply follow the workout instructions.

Workout: Following the **Virtue Level Warm-up**, increase intensity to your recovery pace (base pace RPE minus one) as you pray the Rosary during a 30-minute workout. For some exercisers, the warm-up pace and the recovery pace are essentially the same. Transition to the **Virtue Level Cool-down** during the last 5 minutes.

Journal entry: Log your workout in your journal.

Workout 3 – Base pace training (30 minutes total time):

Focus: Use this steady state workout to practice meditation.

Note: There are no graphics for base pace training workouts in the Virtue Level.   Refer to the base pace training graphic in the Power Level, or simply follow the workout instructions.

Workout: After the **Virtue Level Warm-up**, increase intensity to your base pace (RPE of 4-5), and pray the Rosary during a 30-minute workout. Transition to the **Virtue Level Cool-down** during the last 5 minutes.

Journal entry: Log the workout in your journal.

Workout 4 - Base Pace Training (30 minutes total time):

Focus: This is the first day that you will increase frequency to four days per week.   Modify the RPE and/or duration as needed to allow your body to adapt to the fourth weekly workout. Watch for symptoms of overtraining.

Workout: After the **Virtue Level Warm-up**, increase intensity to your base pace (RPE of 4-5), and try some of the ideas for **unstructured time**. The workout duration goal is 30 minutes, including warm-up and the **Virtue Level Cool-down**

Journal entry: Log your workout in your journal.

"Contemplating the scenes of the Rosary in union with Mary is a means of learning from her to "read" Christ, to discover his secrets and to understand his message."
- Pope John Paul II, Apostolic Letter, Rosary of the Virgin Mary

---

Virtue Level Week 2

Spiritual Component: Finish your study of the Gospel of Mark.

Workout 1 – Intervals (30 minutes total time):

Focus: By now you should be able to complete all 5 intervals at base pace RPE + 1. Continue your efforts toward the new goal of completing five intervals at base pace RPE + 2.

Meditation is a quest and a journey. Some days you will find inspiration and other days you'll struggle to focus on the mysteries. Just as regular workouts improve your physical fitness, regular meditation and study of Sacred Scripture will improve your spiritual fitness.

Workout: After the **Virtue Level Warm-up**, increase intensity to your base pace (RPE of 4-5), and pray the Rosary while completing five intervals. Transition to the **Virtue Level**

Cool-down at the end of the Rosary. (Refer to the graphic for Week 1, Workout 1)

Journal entry: Log your workout in your journal.

Workout 2 – Recovery (30 minutes total time):

Focus: Recovery workouts offer an opportunity to meditate during a relaxed exercise pace.

Workout: Following the **Virtue Level Warm-up**, increase intensity to your recovery pace (base pace RPE minus one) as you pray the Rosary during a 30-minute workout. Transition to the **Virtue Level Cool-down** during the last 5 minutes.

Journal entry: Log your workout in your journal.

Workout 3 – Base Pace Training (30 minutes total time):

Workout: After the **Virtue Level Warm-up**, increase intensity to your base pace (RPE of 4-5), and pray the Rosary during a 30-minute workout. Transition to the **Virtue Level Cool-down** during the last 5 minutes.

Journal entry: Log your workout in your journal.

Workout 4 - Base Pace Training (30 minutes total time):

Workout: After the **Virtue Level Warm-up**, increase intensity to your base pace (RPE of 4-5), and include some of the suggestions for **unstructured time** during a 30-minute workout. Transition to the **Virtue Level Cool-down** during the last 5 minutes.

Journal entry: Log your workout in your journal.

"In the final analysis, what is sport if not a form of education for the body? This education is closely related to morality." (Pope Pius XII, The Sporting Ideal, Rome, May 20, 1945)

Virtue Level Week 3 (Peak Week)

Spiritual Component: This week you'll begin to study of the Gospel of Luke.

Workout 1 – Intervals (30 minutes total time):

Focus: Keep challenging yourself to work a little harder during each interval workout. Remember to diligently study and ponder the Gospels. Simply reading them is certainly beneficial, but you'll learn so much more through a guided study.

Workout: After the **Virtue Level Warm-up**, increase intensity to your base pace (RPE of 4-5), and pray the Rosary while completing five intervals. Transition to the **Virtue Level Cool-down** at the end of the Rosary. (Refer to the graphic for Week 1, Workout 1)

Journal entry: Log the workout in your journal.

Workout 2 – Recovery (30 minutes total time):

Workout: Following the **Virtue Level Warm-up**, increase intensity to your recovery pace (base pace RPE minus one) as you pray the Rosary during a 30-minute workout. Transition to the **Virtue Level Cool-down** during the last 5 minutes.

Journal entry: Log your workout in your journal.

Workout 3 - Intervals (30 minutes total time):

Focus: If you're not feeling up to two interval workouts in one week, complete as many intervals as you can then transition to base pace for the rest of the workout.

Workout: After the **Virtue Level Warm-up**, increase intensity to your base pace (RPE of 4-5), and pray the Rosary while completing five intervals. Transition to the **Virtue Level Cool-down** at the end of the Rosary. (Refer to the graphic for Week 1, Workout 1)

Journal entry: Log your workout in your journal. Record as many details as possible.

Workout 4 - Recovery (30 minutes total time):

Workout: Following the **Virtue Level Warm-up**, increase intensity to your recovery pace (base pace RPE minus one) and include **unstructured time** ideas during a 30-minute workout. Transition to the **Virtue Level Cool-down** during the last 5 minutes.

Journal entry: Log your workout in your journal.

"The prayer of the Rosary is perfect because of the praises it offers, the lessons it teaches, the graces it obtains, and the victories it achieves." - Pope Benedict XV

Virtue Level Week 4 (Recovery Week)

<u>Spiritual Component:</u> Continue your study of the Gospel of Luke.

Workout 1 – Recovery (30 minutes):

<u>Focus:</u> Try a different mode of exercise to keep things fresh. If you normally jog or run, try rollerblading. If you ride a stationary bike, try the stair stepper. If you exercise outside, vary your usual route. A new mode of exercise may require a decrease in RPE and duration.

<u>Workout:</u> Following the **Virtue Level Warm-up**, increase intensity to your recovery pace (base pace RPE minus one) and pray the Rosary during a 30-minute workout. Transition to the **Virtue Level Cool-down** during the last 5 minutes.

<u>Journal entry</u>: Log your workout in your journal.

Workout 2 – Base Pace Training (30 minutes total time):

<u>Focus:</u> During the cool-down, think of a good deed you can do today. Remember that you're learning to <u>live</u> the message of the Gospels you've been studying.

<u>Workout:</u> After the **Virtue Level Warm-up**, increase intensity to your base pace (RPE of 4-5), and pray the Rosary during a 30-minute workout. When you finish the Rosary, transition to the **Virtue Level Cool-down**.

<u>Journal entry</u>: Log your workout in your journal.

Workout 3 – Recovery (30 minutes total time):

<u>Focus:</u> Invite a friend or family member to accompany you today. Pray the Rosary together, discuss your Bible study or just enjoy each other's company. If you can't find a willing exercise partner, take advantage of one who is always with you — your guardian angel. Ask your guardian angel to pray the Rosary with you, and listen for your angel's guidance today.

<u>Workout:</u> Following the **Virtue Level Warm-up**, increase intensity to your recovery pace (base pace RPE minus one) as you pray the Rosary during a 30-minute workout. Transition to the **Virtue Level Cool-down** during the last 5 minutes.

<u>Journal entry</u>: Log your workout in your journal.

Workout 4 – Base Pace Training (30 minutes total time):

<u>Workout:</u> After the **Virtue Level Warm-up**, increase intensity to your base pace (RPE of

4-5), and include some of the suggestions for **unstructured time** during a 30-minute workout. Transition to the **Virtue Level Cool-down** during the last 5 minutes.

Journal entry: Log your workout in your journal.

Congratulations! You have completed the Virtue Level of The Rosary Workout™.

"Among all the devotions approved by the Church, none has been so favored by so many miracles as the Rosary devotion." - Pope Pius IX

Virtue Level Graduation Requirements

You are ready to move on to the Dominion Level if you have met the following conditions:

1. You have exercised 4 days each week for 4 continuous weeks.
2. You are able to complete 5 intervals at base pace RPE + 2
3. You have no symptoms of overtraining.
4. You have completed an in-depth study of at least one gospel.
5a. If you have not met the conditions above, consider extra study and/or workouts before you progress to the Dominion Level. If you struggle with the workouts, continue building on the progress you've made so far until you are able to meet the frequency, duration and intensity goals above. If intervals are too challenging, make sure that you're not trying to push yourself past your limits. Remember, the workout descriptions are a goal, not a requirement. Likewise, if adding an extra day or extra time to your workouts is too much, then give yourself a few extra weeks to meet the Virtue Level goals. You may want to re-evaluate the feasibility of adding extra workout duration or frequency. Modify the suggested workouts to meet your personal time constraints.
5b. If you have not had time to begin an in-depth study of the gospels, then mark a date on your calendar to start. It may take several months to study all four gospels, and that's fine. The important thing is to set aside some time a few days each week to devote to Bible study.
6. Reward yourself for reaching your goal.
7. Don't forget to pray to the Choir of Virtues (and any saints to whom you prayed for intercession) to thank them for their assistance in helping you complete this level.

Virtue Level Completion Assignments:

For the Soul: Continue your monthly commitment to the Sacrament of Confession. Buy or borrow a copy of the Catechism of the Catholic Church (CCC). Ensure you have the most recent edition. Ask the DRE (Director of Religious Education) or RCIA coordinator at your parish if there are copies available for you to borrow. Browse through the Table of Contents or Index and pick a few topics to study or review. Several Catholic sites publish the Catechism online.

For the Body: Turn off the TV or computer for 15-30 minutes and read something. Try this 3-5 times a week. It's important to keep your mind healthy, as well as your body.

Dominion Level Workouts:
Third Intermediate Level (4 weeks)

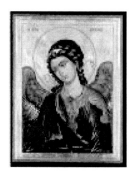

Prayer to the **Choir of Dominions:**

By the intercession of St. Michael and the celestial Choir of Dominions may the Lord give us grace to govern our senses and overcome any unruly passions. Amen.

-From the Chaplet of St. Michael the Archangel

Pray to the Choir of Dominions and your own guardian angel for help to complete this level.

Dominion Level Summary and Goals:

During the Dominion Level, you will continue to improve fitness by increasing the duration of intervals and the frequency of interval workouts. You'll finish the study of all four Gospels.

There are two types of interval training in the Dominion Level. The previous intervals in the Power and Virtue Level begin with the Glory Be and end with the Our Father of a given decade. From now on these will be called "short intervals," and are still included in the program. I'll also introduce a new type of interval called "long intervals". During long intervals, the increased pace is held through the ten Hail Mary's of a given decade (about 2 minutes). Of course, this is a goal which will require time and effort to master.

It will be a challenge to meditate while completing the long intervals as you'll tend focus more on the physical discomfort. The Rosary prayers can be used for encouragement: "I can keep going through the next two Hail Mary's," for instance. I certainly don't advocate continuing an interval past the point of exhaustion, but I do encourage you to exceed your comfort level a bit. You can look to the mysteries themselves to help you overcome the difficulty of this challenge. The Sorrowful Mysteries are particularly inspiring in this application. Learning to meditate during a tough physical effort is a skill that you will draw on during life's difficulties.

Dominion Level Goals:

1. Increase the duration of intervals (up to 2 minutes).

2. Increase the frequency of interval workouts.

3. Maintain exercise frequency at 4 days per week.

<u>Note</u>: If you cannot exercise four times a week, you can still complete the Dominion Level. Accomplish the workouts in order, at a frequency of three per week. <u>Specific instructions are not included for these modifications.</u>

4. Finish an in-depth study of the four Gospels

After completing the Dominion Level you should be able to:

1. Pray the Rosary during exercise for 30 minutes, 4 days each week.

2. Complete 3 long intervals during a workout (about 2 minutes each).

3. Attain a deeper understanding of the four Gospels.

Spiritual Component for the Dominion Level:

You'll spend the first week finishing your study of the Gospel of Luke. The remaining three weeks are devoted to studying the Gospel of John. Refer to the section on **Bible Translations and Study Guides**, if needed.

Exercise Components for the Dominion Level:

Frequency: 4 days per week

Duration: 30 minutes total time for each workout

Intensity:

Warm-up and Cool-down: Easy to Moderate (3-4 on RPE scale)

Base pace: Moderate to Somewhat Hard (4-5 on RPE scale)

Intervals: Base pace RPE + 2 (short intervals) or base pace RPE + 1 (long intervals)

Recovery: Base pace RPE minus 1

Mode: Any type of rhythmic aerobic exercise (walking, biking, etc.)

Dominion Level Warm-up: The Dominion Level warm-up is the same throughout all the workouts in this level and is therefore listed only once. As you begin the physical portion of the warm-up, you should also "warm-up" spiritually. Begin exercise at an RPE of 3-4 while you say a short prayer to the Holy Spirit, your patron saint or the Blessed Mother asking for help in reaching your physical and spiritual goals. Decide on a Rosary intention based on your own needs or those of others. The warm-up should last at least 5 minutes. You are ready to begin your workout with the opening prayer of the Rosary, The Apostles' Creed.

Dominion Level Cool-down: The Dominion Level cool-down is also the same throughout all the workouts in this level. Slow your pace to an RPE of 3-4 for about 5 minutes. Use this time to reflect on the mysteries, think of a good deed you can do today, or enjoy your surroundings and the feeling of accomplishment in finishing your workout.

Stretch: If time allows after your workout, take a few minutes to stretch the major muscle groups you worked during exercise. If you don't have time to stretch, try to fit in a stretching session later in the day or at least 2-3 times each week.

Dominion Level Week 1

Spiritual Component: Finish your study of the Gospel of Luke. Refer to the section on **Bible Translations and Study Guides**, if needed.

Workout 1 - Long Intervals (30 minutes):

Focus: This workout is different from previous interval workouts. From now on, I'll refer to intervals the way they were presented in the Power and Virtue Level as "short intervals," meaning that the interval begins at the Glory Be and ends with the Our Father of a given decade. Today we'll begin a new type of interval -- "long intervals". The prayers used to mark the duration of the long intervals are the ten Hail Mary's of a given decade. The long interval pace is base pace RPE + 1. Refer to the graphic on the next page to understand how the intervals and recovery periods are incorporated with the Rosary prayers.

You may struggle with meditation during the long intervals. Refer to the Dominion Level summary for suggestions.

Workout: After the **Dominion Level Warm-up**, increase intensity to your base pace (RPE of 4-5) and begin praying the Rosary.

The **first long interval** begins with the first Hail Mary of the second decade. Increase your pace slightly to base pace RPE + 1. This is not an all-out effort but a pace you can sustain for about 2 minutes. This is a good time to use the "talk test" to judge RPE by saying the prayers out loud. Your goal is to maintain the increased pace through all 10 Hail Mary's. The recovery period begins with the Glory Be at the end of the 2nd decade and continues through the Fatima Prayer, 3rd mystery announcement, 3rd decade of Hail Mary's, 4th mystery announcement and Our Father. The recovery pace is base pace RPE minus 1. (Note that this is your interval RPE minus 2.)

The **second long interval** begins with the 4th decade of Hail Mary's. Again, the goal is to maintain the interval pace through all 10 Hail Mary's, but you can skip or shorten this interval. Recover during the rest of the Rosary, then transition to the **Dominion Level Cool-down** .

Note: Resume your base pace during recovery when you're ready to do so.

Journal entry: Log your workout in your journal. Since this is a new type of interval workout, the more details you enter, the better your ability to plan future workouts. Include notes about any struggles, revelations or thoughts you experienced during your Rosary meditation.

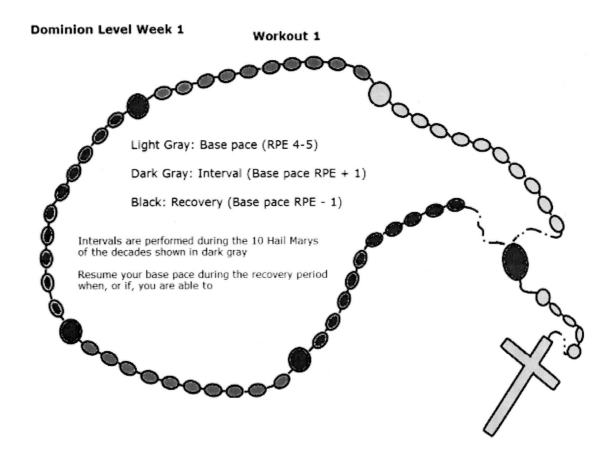

Dominion Level Week 1

Workout 1

Light Gray: Base pace (RPE 4-5)

Dark Gray: Interval (Base pace RPE + 1)

Black: Recovery (Base pace RPE - 1)

Intervals are performed during the 10 Hail Marys
of the decades shown in dark gray

Resume your base pace during the recovery period
when, or if, you are able to

Workout 2 - Recovery (30 minutes total time):

Workout: After the **Dominion Level Warm-up**, increase intensity to your recovery pace (base pace RPE minus one) as you pray the Rosary during a 30-minute workout. Transition to the **Dominion Level Cool-down** during the last 5 minutes of the workout.

Journal entry: Log your workout in your journal.

Workout 3 – Base Pace Training (30 minutes total time):

Workout: After the **Dominion Level Warm-up**, increase intensity to your base pace (**RPE** of 4-5), and pray the Rosary during a 30-minute workout. Transition to the **Dominion Level Cool-down** during the last 5 minutes of the workout.

Journal entry: Log your workout in your journal.

Workout 4 – Base Pace Training (30 minutes total time):

Focus: Include **unstructured time** ideas today as an alternative to praying the Rosary.

Workout: After the **Dominion Level Warm-up**, increase intensity to your base pace (RPE of 4-5), and include **unstructured time** ideas during a 30-minute workout. Transition to the **Dominion Level Cool-down** during the last 5 minutes of the workout.

Journal entry: Log your workout in your journal.

"Blessed are we if we are faithful in reciting that very popular and splendid prayer, the Rosary, which is a kind of measured spelling out of our feelings of affection in the invocation: Hail Mary, Hail Mary, Hail Mary... Our life will be a fortunate one if it is interwoven with this garland of roses, with this circlet of praises to Mary, to the mysteries of her Divine Son!" -Pope Paul VI

Dominion Level Week 2

Spiritual Component: Begin a study of the Gospel of John.

Workout 1 – Long Intervals (30 minutes total time):

Focus: Today you will repeat the long interval workout that you did last week.

Workout: After the **Dominion Level Warm-up**, increase intensity to your base pace (RPE of 4-5) and begin praying the Rosary. Complete two long intervals during the second and fourth decades. Refer to the detailed instructions and graphic for Week 1, Workout 1. Transition to the **Dominion Level Cool-down** after your finish the Rosary.

Journal entry: Log your workout in your journal.

Workout 2 – Recovery (30 minutes):

Focus: Use this easy workout to practice meditative Rosary prayer. Reflect on your Gospel study for a deeper understanding of the mysteries.
Workout: After the **Dominion Level Warm-up**, increase intensity to your recovery pace (base pace RPE minus one) as you pray the Rosary during a 30-minute workout. Transition to the **Dominion Level Cool-down** during the last 5 minutes of the workout.

Journal entry: Log your workout in your journal.

Workout 3 – Short Intervals (30 minutes total time):

Focus: Today is a short interval workout. Refer to your journal entries from the Virtue Level to recall the details of your last short interval workout.

As always, use the rhythm of the interval workouts to emphasize the transition between Rosary decades and the division of meditation periods. Lift your mind and heart to heaven during the intervals and return to focused meditation in the recovery periods.

Workout: After completing the **Dominion Level Warm-up**, increase intensity to base pace (RPE of 4-5), and pray the Rosary while completing five short intervals at base pace RPE + 2. Transition to the **Dominion Level Cool-down** after your finish the Rosary.

Journal entry: Log your workout in your journal.

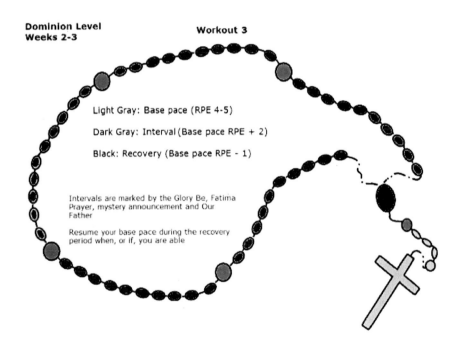

Dominion Level Weeks 2-3

Workout 3

Light Gray: Base pace (RPE 4-5)

Dark Gray: Interval (Base pace RPE + 2)

Black: Recovery (Base pace RPE - 1)

Intervals are marked by the Glory Be, Fatima Prayer, mystery announcement and Our Father

Resume your base pace during the recovery period when, or if, you are able

Workout 4 – Recovery (30 minutes total time)

Workout: After the **Dominion Level Warm-up**, increase intensity to your recovery pace (base pace RPE minus one) and include **unstructured time** ideas during a 30-minute workout. Transition to the **Dominion Level Cool-down** during the last 5 minutes of the workout.

Journal entry: Log your workout in your journal.

Exercise is powerful preventative medicine. It helps prevent premature death, heart disease, high blood pressure, diabetes and other diseases.

Spiritual Component: Continue your study of the Gospel of John.

Workout 1 – Long Intervals (30 minutes):

Focus: Today is a long interval workout, and you'll add one more for a total of three.

Workout: After the **Dominion Level Warm-up**, increase intensity to your base pace (RPE of 4-5) and begin praying the Rosary.

The **first long interval** is marked by the first decade of Hail Mary's. Begin recovery with the Glory Be and continue through the Our Father at the beginning of the 3rd decade. Interval pace is base pace RPE + 1 and recovery pace is base pace RPE minus 1.

The **second long interval** is marked by the third decade of Hail Mary's. Recover until the end of the Our Father at the beginning of the 5th decade.

The **third long interval** is marked by the fifth decade of Hail Mary's. The recovery period is short -- Glory Be, Fatima Prayer and Hail Holy Queen, so you may need a longer cool-down than usual. Transition to the **Dominion Level Cool-down** after your finish the Rosary.

Journal entry:
Log your workout in your journal. Record pertinent details to help you plan your next interval workout.

Dominion Level Week 3   Workout 1

Light Gray: Base pace (RPE 4-5)

Dark Gray: Interval (Base pace RPE + 1)

Black: Recovery (Base pace RPE - 1)

Intervals are performed during the 10 Hail Marys of the decades shown in dark gray

Resume your base pace during the recovery period when, or if, you are able to

Workout 2 Recovery (30 min.):

Focus:
Don't skip these key recovery workouts or try to increase the suggested RPE.

Workout: After the **Dominion Level Warm-up**, increase intensity to your recovery pace (base pace RPE minus one) as you pray the Rosary during a 30-minute workout. When you finish the Rosary, transition to the **Dominion Level Cool-down**.

Journal entry: Log your workout in your journal.

Workout 3 – Short Intervals (30 minutes total time):

Workout: After completing the **Dominion Level Warm-up**, increase intensity to base pace (RPE of 4-5), and pray the Rosary while completing five short intervals at base pace RPE + 2. Transition to the **Dominion Level Cool-down** after your finish the Rosary. Refer to the graphic for Week 2, Workout 3.

Journal entry: Log your workout in your journal.

Workout 4 – Recovery (30 minutes total time)

Focus: Include **unstructured time** ideas today as an alternative to praying the Rosary.

Workout: After the **Dominion Level Warm-up**, increase intensity to your recovery pace (base pace RPE minus one) and include **unstructured time** ideas during a 30-minute workout. Transition to the **Dominion Level Cool-down** during the last 5 minutes.

Journal entry: Log your workout in your journal.

"Take care of your body with steadfast fidelity. The soul must see through these eyes alone, and if they are dim, the whole world is clouded." -Johann Wolfgang von Goethe

---

Dominion Level Week 4 (Recovery Week)

Spiritual Component: Finish your study of the Gospel of John.

Workout 1 – Base Pace Training (30 minutes):

Focus: During the cool-down, think of a good deed that you can do today.

Workout: After the **Dominion Level Warm-up**, increase intensity to your base pace (RPE of 4-5), and pray the Rosary during a 30-minute workout. Transition to the **Dominion Level Cool-down** during the last 5 minutes of the workout.

Journal entry: Log your workout in your journal.

Workout 2 - Recovery (30 minutes total time):

Focus: Take it easy today as a recovery workout. Invite a friend or family member to accompany you during your workout, or talk to your guardian angel.

Workout: After the **Dominion Level Warm-up**, increase intensity to your recovery pace (base pace RPE minus one) as you pray the Rosary during a 30-minute workout. When you finish the Rosary, transition to the **Dominion Level Cool-down**.

Journal entry: Log your workout in your journal.

Workout 3 - Base Pace Training (30 minutes total time):

Focus: Try a different mode of exercise to keep things fresh. If you usually swim, then walk or jog today. Vary your usual route or try a new piece of equipment at the gym.

Workout: After the **Dominion Level Warm-up**, increase intensity to your base pace (RPE of 4-5), and pray the Rosary during a 30-minute workout. Transition to the **Dominion Level Cool-down** during the last 5 minutes of the workout.

Journal entry: Log your workout in your journal.

Workout 4 – Stretching (30 minutes total time)

No structured workout today. Instead, warm-up for 5-10 minutes and spend about 15-30 minutes gently stretching. Optional: Include **unstructured time** ideas as you stretch.

Congratulations! You have completed the Dominion Level of The Rosary Workout™ as well as the Intermediate Level of the program.

No rest is worth anything except the rest that is earned. -Jean Paul

---

Dominion Level Graduation Requirements

You are ready to move on to the Advanced Level if you have met the following conditions:

1. You have exercised for 30 minutes, 4 days each week for 4 continuous weeks.
2. You are able to complete 3 long intervals (about 2 minutes each).
3. You have no symptoms of overtraining.
4. You have completed your in-depth study of the gospels.
5a. If you have not met the conditions above, consider extra study and/or workouts before you progress to the Advanced Series and the Throne Level. If you struggle with the workouts, continue building on the progress you've made so far until you are able to meet the frequency, duration and intensity goals above. If intervals are too challenging, make sure that you're not trying to push yourself past your limits. Remember that the workout descriptions are a goal, not a requirement. Take as much time as you need to finish the Dominion Level.
5b. If you still have not had time to begin an in-depth study of the gospels, then you may find a Scriptural Rosary booklet helpful until you can find room in your schedule for Bible study. Although not a replacement for actual study of the Bible, it can help you with meditation.

Read through the Bible references before your workout, or pray the Rosary using the booklet during a quiet time when you're not exercising.

6. Reward yourself for reaching your goal.

7. Don't forget to pray to the Choir of Dominions (and any saints to whom you prayed for intercession) to thank them for their assistance in helping you complete this level.

Dominion Level Completion Assignments:

For the Soul: Don't forget to go to Confession! Your assignment is to learn more about a new saint. If you were named after a saint and don't know much about him/her, then do some research. Perhaps you could read about the patron saint of your job (St. Isidore is the patron saint of farmers, for instance) or a hobby (St. Hubert is the patron saint of hunters). There are several fascinating modern-day saints such as St. Pio (known as Padre Pio), St. Therese of Lisieux, St. Gianna Molla, Blessed Pier Giorgio Frassatti, Blessed Teresa of Calcutta (Mother Teresa), etc.

For the Body: Add some resistance or weight training to your weekly workouts. Join a gym or buy a few sets of dumbbells, stretch cords or a medicine ball at a sporting goods or discount store. If you are new to weight training, consider hiring a personal trainer to ensure you use proper form and avoid injury. Interview trainers and ask for the trainer's credentials, experience and references. State your needs clearly and ask for a *specific plan* to meet your goals. Talk to some of the trainer's clients before making a final decision. If your budget is a factor, many trainers offer group sessions. Ask to join an existing group, or recruit friends or family members to share the expense. Another option is to hire a trainer to come to your home. Since gyms take a huge cut of a trainer's pay, you may be able to save money by hiring an independent trainer. If you live near a college or university that has an Exercise Physiology department, ask if the students offer personal training services. Perhaps you can save up for a few personal training sessions as a reward for completing a level of The Rosary Workout™.

Note: You may not want to progress to the Advanced Series, and that is perfectly fine. If you only have time to exercise 3 times a week or no more than 30 minutes at a time, you can still maintain a healthy level of fitness and even train for an athletic event such as a 5k run/walk or triathlon. Read through the Advanced Series for ideas on how to add occasional challenges to your workouts. Try to fit in a long recovery workout when you have a little extra time. In any case, continue your habit of regular exercise. You've worked hard to establish an above-average fitness level.

Do realize that you should continue to progress in Mary's School of the Rosary. If you haven't finished an in-depth study of the gospels, continue reading, studying and reflecting on the words and examples of Christ. Read through the advanced spiritual components and the end-of-level homework assignments for ideas on how to improve your spiritual fitness.

Advanced Series

The Advanced Series is the culmination of The Rosary Workout™ program. The skills and knowledge you've acquired are brought together so that you can "graduate" to designing your own physical and spiritual fitness program. You still have much to learn, but you will have achieved a high level of fitness and a lifelong devotion to the Rosary.
"Therefore, glorify God in your body." (1 Corinthians 6:20)

There are three levels in the Advanced Series: **Throne**, **Cherubim** and **Seraphim**. This series assumes that you are at the advanced level in both physical fitness and in Mary's School of praying the Rosary. Refer to the definitions of the **advanced exerciser** and the **Advanced Level of Mary's School**, if needed.

Please try to follow the plan as much as possible. The periodized workouts are designed to prevent injury and overtraining.

The Advanced Series requires exercise at least 4-5 days a week for 45 minutes or more. (A 3-day-per-week modification is outlined but does not include specific workouts.) This program is ideal for athletes or those who would like to train for an event such as a marathon, triathlon, 5k/10k race, cycling event, etc. However, anyone who wants to increase overall fitness or who enjoys a challenge will benefit from the Advanced Level workouts.

It is important to work up to this level. If you are new to The Rosary Workout™ program, do not jump to the Advanced Series simply because you want to try the hardest workouts first. Even if you are an advanced exerciser or a competitive athlete, consider that praying the Rosary and meditating while you exercise is a skill that must be practiced and doesn't come naturally. I highly recommend that you modify your current workout routine to include two or three Beginner workouts each week. Increase the duration and suggested RPE as needed, and follow the spiritual exercises until you are comfortable with Rosary meditation during steady-state exercise. If you are not familiar with interval training, then try a few of the intermediate workouts so that you fully understand how the Rosary prayers mark the intervals and recovery periods.

You've worked very hard to attain this advanced level of fitness. It's important that you apply this same dedication to your study of the Rosary and your practice in meditation.

Advanced students of the Rosary continually strive to practice the virtues portrayed by each of the mysteries as they continue to study and ponder the Word of God.

Jesus Himself praises such accomplishment in the Parable of the Sower:

"But the seed sown on rich soil is the one who hears the Word and understands it, who indeed bears fruit and yields a hundred or sixty or thirtyfold." (Matthew 13:23)

Throne Level Workouts: First Advanced Level (4 weeks)

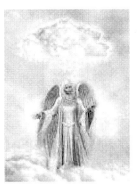

Prayer to the **Choir of Thrones:**

By the intercession of St. Michael and the celestial Choir of Thrones may the Lord infuse into our hearts a true and sincere spirit of humility. Amen.

-From the Chaplet of St. Michael the Archangel

Pray to the Choir of Thrones and your guardian angel for assistance in completing this level.

Throne Level Summary and Goals:

During the Throne Level, you will improve fitness by increasing the frequency of short intervals and the duration of long intervals. The Rating of Perceived Exertion (RPE) levels are increased from those in the intermediate workouts. To grow spiritually, you'll add to your resources for Rosary meditation.

As an advanced exerciser, you have a lot of control over your body and you have the mental willpower to push past physical limits. As an advanced student of the Rosary, you have spent countless hours studying and pondering the mysteries. You have the mental willpower to concentrate on each mystery and overcome distractions. The Throne Level will require the combination of physical strength and mental willpower to practice Rosary meditation during very challenging workouts.

Note: Since you'll pray the Rosary at least three times a week during your workouts, you can join the Confraternity of the Holy Rosary. Members pledge to pray all 15 traditional mysteries each week. (The addition of the Luminous mysteries is encouraged, but not required.) This organization can be traced back to St. Dominic, the great Rosary saint. There are many powerful promises, benefits and indulgences for members of this confraternity, and there's no cost to join. Learn more at their website: **www.rosary-center.org**

Throne Level Goals:

1. Increase the total number of short intervals

2. Increase the duration of long intervals

3. Maintain frequency at 4 days per week.

Note: If you cannot exercise more than 3 times a week, you can still complete this level. Accomplish the workouts in order, but do 3 workouts each week. The 4th workout for Week 1 will become the 1ˢᵗ workout for Week 2, etc. Obviously, this will take more than 4 weeks, and the peak and recovery weeks won't line up. Modify the program to fit your schedule. You should increase the duration of the Throne Level workouts to 40-60 minutes so that you maintain the fitness level you reached during the Dominion Level. Refer to your journal to help you plan the workouts. <u>Specific instructions are not included for these modifications</u>.

4. Incorporate the advanced workout cycle: A short interval workout, followed by long-interval workout, followed by a recovery day.

5. Expand your study of the Rosary and the mysteries

After completing the Throne Level you should be able to:

1. Pray the Rosary during exercise for 30-50 minutes, 4 days each week.

2. Complete 10 short intervals.

3. Complete 2 double long intervals (maintain an interval pace while praying 2 decades of the Rosary).

4. Improve Rosary meditation through reading the Bible, papal documents, writings of the saints, or other sources.

Spiritual Component for the Throne Level:

You have many options to expand your knowledge of the Rosary mysteries as an advanced student of Mary's School. One is to continue to study the Bible. You might concentrate on the rest of the New Testament (Acts of the Apostles, Epistles and Revelation) to learn about the Early Church and the spread of Christianity. Or, you can study the Old Testament to learn how events, prophecies and psalms are fulfilled by Jesus in the Gospels and the mysteries of the Rosary. Refer to the section on **Bible Translations and Study Guides** for more information.

Another option is to study the works of great saints, especially those who were Rosary advocates. Books written by St. Louis de Montfort are insightful and easy to read and understand. If you are up to the challenge, the works of St. Thomas Aquinas and St. Teresa of Avila are fascinating. Studying the heroic martyrs from the era of Christian persecution by the Romans can inspire anyone to learn to live the gospels. Modern-day saints offer excellent examples of how to live a holy life in our current times. There are plenty of books about recent saints such as Blessed Teresa of Calcutta (Mother Teresa), St. Pio (Padre Pio), St. Gianna Molla, St. Maximilian Kolbe, St. Faustina, Blessed Pier Giorgio Frassati, and St. Teresa of Lisieux.

You might be interested in studying papal documents on the Rosary, written by various popes throughout history. There is a wealth of wisdom and knowledge in the Apostolic Letter, *Rosary of the Virgin Mary*, by Pope John Paul II. Pope Benedict XVI has also written about the Rosary and other important topics. *Mary ~ Ever Virgin, Full of Grace: A study of Papal*

Encyclicals is a compilation of twelve documents that focus on Mary and the Rosary. It is available at **www.BezalelBooks.com** under the Mary Study link.

Search for documents on the Rosary at the Vatican's website: **www.vatican.va**

During the Advanced Series, choose one of the suggested resources (or something else you're interested in), and study or read it for the next four weeks.

Exercise Components for the Throne Level:

Frequency: 4 days per week

Duration: 30-50 minutes each workout

Intensity:

Warm-up and Cool-down: Moderate to Somewhat Hard (4-5 on RPE scale)

Base pace: Somewhat Hard to Hard (5-6 on RPE scale)

Short intervals: Base pace RPE + 2

Long intervals: Base pace RPE + 1

Recovery: Base pace RPE minus 1

Note: Adjust the RPE suggestions above, based on your current fitness level

Mode: Any type of rhythmic aerobic exercise (walking, biking, etc.) Vary your mode of exercise frequently to prevent boredom and improve fitness. Triathlons (bike, run and swim) are fun and challenging. If you are training for a running event such as a 10k or marathon, try to incorporate some cycling workouts to minimize the impact of constant running.

Throne Level Warm-up: The Throne Level warm-up is the same throughout all the workouts in this level and is therefore listed only once. As you begin the physical portion of the warm-up, you should also "warm-up" spiritually. Begin exercise at an RPE of 4-5 while you say a short prayer to the Holy Spirit, your patron saint or the Blessed Mother asking for help in reaching your physical and spiritual goals. Decide on a Rosary intention based on your own needs or those of others. The warm-up should last at least 5 minutes and perhaps longer if indicated in the workout instructions. You are ready to begin your workout with the opening prayer of the Rosary, The Apostles' Creed.

Throne Level Cool-down: The Throne Level cool-down is also the same throughout all the workouts in this level. Slow your pace to an RPE of 4-5 for at least 5 minutes. Use this time to reflect on the mysteries, think of a good deed you can do today, or enjoy your surroundings and the great feeling of accomplishment in finishing your workout.

Stretch: If time allows after your workout, take a few minutes to stretch the major muscle groups you worked during exercise. If you don't have time to stretch, try to fit in a stretching session later in the day or at least 2-3 times each week.

Throne Level Week 1

Spiritual Component: Begin reading your chosen resource.

Workout 1 – Short Intervals (35-40 minutes total time):

Focus: Today you'll accomplish 6-7 intervals. (For the additional intervals, you will pray part of a second Rosary.) This will slightly increase the workout duration to a total of 35-40 minutes. By now, you should be able to do five short intervals (Glory Be through Our Father) at an intensity of base pace RPE + 2. Refer to your journal entries for the Dominion Level to determine your base pace and the number, length and RPE of your usual short intervals.

The graphics (one for each Rosary) follow the workout instructions and clarify the additional intervals and recovery periods and how they are incorporated with the Rosary prayers.

As you increase your pace during the interval, allow the corresponding prayers to lift your thoughts to heaven as you praise and glorify the Trinity, ask for God's mercy and transition to the next mystery. During the recovery, return your focus to meditation on the new mystery.

Workout: After completing the **Throne Level Warm-up**, increase intensity to your base pace (RPE of 5-6), and pray the Rosary while completing five short intervals. Interval pace is base pace RPE + 2. Recovery pace is base pace RPE minus one. If you recover before the end of the decade, resume your base pace.

During the sixth interval you will begin a second Rosary. This interval is the same duration as previous intervals, but the marking of the prayers on the Rosary is slightly different because you are transitioning to the second Rosary. Again, it's helpful to refer to the graphic while reading the instructions.

The **6th interval** will begin with the Glory Be at the end of the 5th decade. Increase your usual interval pace as you pray the Glory Be, and Fatima Prayer (you will skip the Hail Holy Queen, marked by the medal in the center of the Rosary, for now). Continue the interval as you announce the first mystery of a new set of mysteries (see note below) and the Our Father, which are marked by the last bead on the pendant chain.

Note: You will not pray the other prayers on the pendant chain (Apostles' Creed and three Hail Mary's) for this second Rosary. The second set of mysteries is simply a different set than those you meditated upon during the first Rosary. For example, if you prayed the first Rosary while meditating on the Joyful Mysteries, then you will pray the second Rosary while meditating on a the Luminous, Sorrowful or Glorious Mysteries, your choice). Of course, you can always repeat the same set of mysteries, especially if you were distracted or had trouble meditating during the first Rosary.

Recover during the 10 Hail Mary's of the first new mystery. Although this is really your 6th decade, it is marked by the first 10 Hail Mary's after the center medal. Resume your base pace RPE when, or if, you are able.

If you're still feeling strong, add an additional interval. This **7th interval** begins with the Glory Be at the end of the first new decade of the second Rosary. It ends, as usual, with the Our Father. Your recovery period is marked by the 10 Hail Mary's of the second decade, followed by the **Throne Level Cool-down**. (Optional: Continue to pray the second Rosary during the cool-down). End with the Hail Holy Queen, even if you did not complete all five decades of the second Rosary

Note 1: Please do not add more than 2 short intervals today. Modify the interval duration or RPE if needed.

Note 2: If you prefer to pray only one Rosary, you can still accomplish the additional intervals without praying a second Rosary. Use a watch or other timing device to determine the duration of each interval and recovery period as you complete the first five intervals while praying the Rosary. During the 6th and 7th intervals, delete the references to the second Rosary and use timing instead. As a guide, the short intervals (Glory Be, Fatima Prayer, mystery announcement and Our Father) usually take about 45-60 seconds to complete. The recovery period (10 Hail Mary's) lasts about 2 minutes.

Journal entry: Log your workout in your journal. Use as many specific details as possible to help you plan future interval workouts.

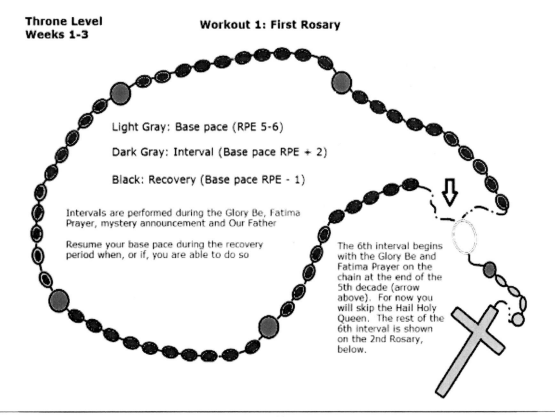

Throne Level
Weeks 1-3

Workout 1: First Rosary

Light Gray: Base pace (RPE 5-6)

Dark Gray: Interval (Base pace RPE + 2)

Black: Recovery (Base pace RPE - 1)

Intervals are performed during the Glory Be, Fatima Prayer, mystery announcement and Our Father

Resume your base pace during the recovery period when, or if, you are able to do so

The 6th interval begins with the Glory Be and Fatima Prayer on the chain at the end of the 5th decade (arrow above). For now you will skip the Hail Holy Queen. The rest of the 6th interval is shown on the 2nd Rosary, below.

Throne Level Week 1

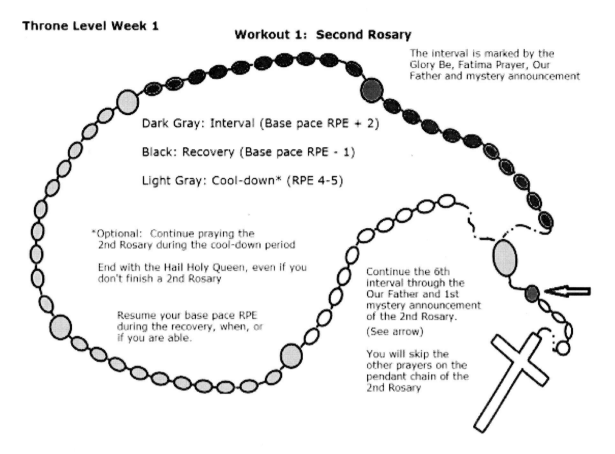

Workout 1: Second Rosary

The interval is marked by the Glory Be, Fatima Prayer, Our Father and mystery announcement

Dark Gray: Interval (Base pace RPE + 2)

Black: Recovery (Base pace RPE - 1)

Light Gray: Cool-down* (RPE 4-5)

*Optional: Continue praying the 2nd Rosary during the cool-down period

End with the Hail Holy Queen, even if you don't finish a 2nd Rosary

Resume your base pace RPE during the recovery, when, or if you are able.

Continue the 6th interval through the Our Father and 1st mystery announcement of the 2nd Rosary. (See arrow)

You will skip the other prayers on the pendant chain of the 2nd Rosary

Workout 2 – Recovery (30 minutes):

Focus: This workout is designed to be easy and serves as an active recovery. Try to plan a recovery workout the day after a high-intensity workout.

Workout: After the **Throne Level Warm-up**, increase intensity to your recovery pace (base pace RPE minus one) as you pray the Rosary during a 30-minute workout. For some exercisers, the warm-up pace and the recovery pace are essentially the same. When you finish the Rosary, transition to the **Throne Level Cool-down**.

Journal entry: Log your workout in your journal.

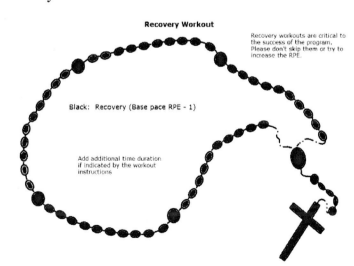

Recovery Workout

Recovery workouts are critical to the success of the program. Please don't skip them or try to increase the RPE.

Black: Recovery (Base pace RPE - 1)

Add additional time duration if indicated by the workout instructions

<u>Note</u>: Refer to this graphic for all recovery workouts in the Advanced Series.

Workout 3 – Long Intervals (30 minutes total time):

Focus: Today's long interval workout is slightly different from those in the intermediate level. The recovery period is shortened in order to increase the overall intensity of the workout. Basically, it's a reversal of the short intervals: You'll maintain the long interval pace (base pace RPE + 1) during the 10 Hail Mary's and recover during the Glory Be, Fatima Prayer, mystery announcement and Our Father, then repeat the long interval during the next 10 Hail Mary's. The goal today is three intervals. Refer to the graphic at the end of the workout to help you visualize how the intervals correspond to the Rosary prayers.

This workout presents a challenge for meditation as you strive to reach the physical goals. Use the mental discipline you apply to exercise to direct your thoughts to the mysteries. This skill takes practice and perseverance.

Workout: After the **Throne Level Warm-up**, increase intensity to your base pace (RPE of 5-6) and begin praying the Rosary.

The **first long interval** is marked by the 2nd decade of Hail Mary's. Increase your pace slightly to base pace RPE + 1. Use the "talk test" to judge RPE by saying the prayers out loud. The recovery period begins with the Glory Be and continues through the Our Father. Slow to base pace RPE minus 1 (or interval RPE minus 2) during this short recovery.

The **second long interval** is marked by the 3rd decade of Hail Mary's. Again, the shorter recovery period starts with the Glory Be and continues through the Our Father.

The **third long interval** is marked by the 4th decade of Hail Mary's. Recover during the Glory Be through the Our Father.

Resume your base pace during the 5th decade and Hail Holy Queen, or use the time for additional recovery. When you finish the Rosary, transition to the **Throne Level Cool-down**.

Journal entry: Log your workout in your journal. Since you're using the Rosary prayers as a timing method for intervals and recovery time, use them as references in your journal. Make sure you include details about the intervals — at what point did you became tired during the interval? How long did it last? When were you able to resume your base pace? When did you feel like you were ready for another interval? Be sure to add notes about any revelations or thoughts you experienced during your Rosary meditation.

Throne Level Week 1

Workout 3

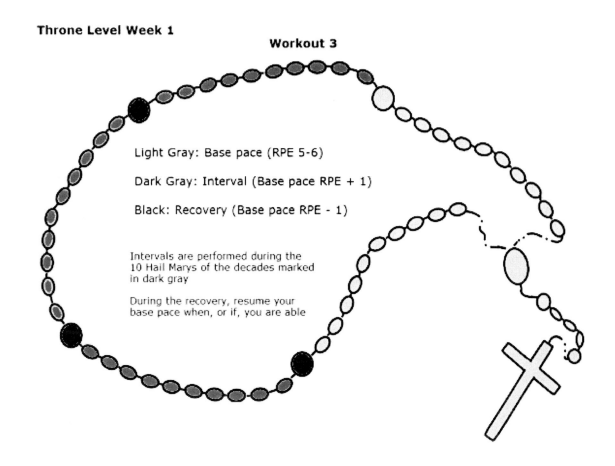

Light Gray: Base pace (RPE 5-6)

Dark Gray: Interval (Base pace RPE + 1)

Black: Recovery (Base pace RPE - 1)

Intervals are performed during the
10 Hail Marys of the decades marked
in dark gray

During the recovery, resume your
base pace when, or if, you are able

Workout 4 – Recovery (30 minutes total time)

Workout: Following the **Throne Level Warm-up**, increase intensity to your recovery pace (base pace RPE minus one), and include **unstructured time** ideas during a 30-minute recovery workout. Transition to the **Throne Level Cool-down** during the last 5 minutes.

Journal entry: Log your workout in your journal.

"The Rosary, as is known to all, is in fact a very excellent means of prayer and meditation in the form of a mystical crown in which the prayers Our Father, Hail Mary, and Glory be to the Father are intertwined with meditation on the greatest mysteries of our Faith and which presents to the mind, like many pictures, the drama of the Incarnation of our Lord and the Redemption." -Pope John XXIII

Spiritual Component: Continue reading the source you've chosen.

Workout 1 – Short Intervals (35-45 minutes total time):

Focus: The number of short intervals increases to 8-9 total. (For the additional intervals, you will pray part of a second Rosary or use timing.) Total workout duration is 35-45 minutes. Refer to Week 1, Workout 1 for the detailed description of this workout.

Workout: After the **Throne Level Warm-up**, increase intensity to your base pace (RPE of 5-6), and pray the first Rosary while completing five short intervals. Continue with the 6th and 7th intervals, as explained in the instructions for Week 1, Workout 1.

The **8th interval** begins with the Glory Be at the end of the second decade of the second Rosary. It ends, with the Our Father. The recovery period is marked by the 10 Hail Mary's of the third decade of the second Rosary.

The **9th interval** begins with the Glory Be at the end of the third decade of the second Rosary and ends with the Our Father. The recovery period is marked by the 10 Hail Mary's of the 4th decade of the second Rosary. Transition to the **Throne Level Cool-down** as you finish praying the second Rosary.

Note 1: End with a Hail Holy Queen, even if you did not complete all five decades of the 2nd Rosary.

Note 2: If you prefer to pray only one Rosary, use the timing method described in Week 1, Workout 1 for the 6th- 9th intervals.

Journal entry: Log your workout in your journal.

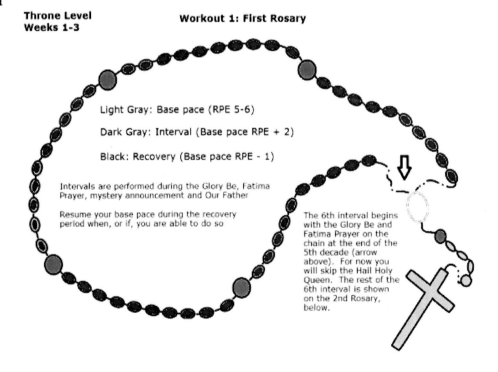

Throne Level Weeks 1-3

Workout 1: First Rosary

Light Gray: Base pace (RPE 5-6)

Dark Gray: Interval (Base pace RPE + 2)

Black: Recovery (Base pace RPE - 1)

Intervals are performed during the Glory Be, Fatima Prayer, mystery announcement and Our Father

Resume your base pace during the recovery period when, or if, you are able to do so

The 6th interval begins with the Glory Be and Fatima Prayer on the chain at the end of the 5th decade (arrow above). For now you will skip the Hail Holy Queen. The rest of the 6th interval is shown on the 2nd Rosary, below.

Throne Level Week 2

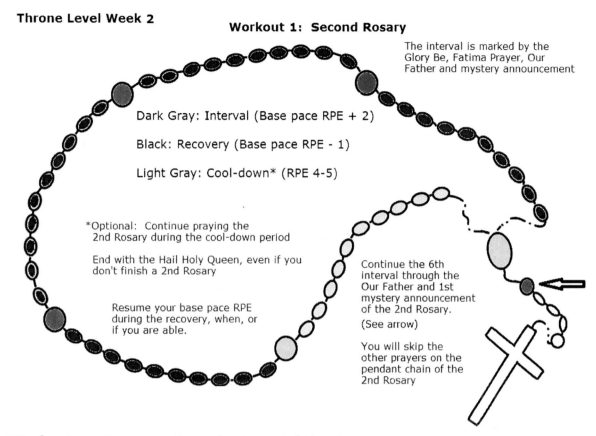

Workout 1: Second Rosary

The interval is marked by the Glory Be, Fatima Prayer, Our Father and mystery announcement

Dark Gray: Interval (Base pace RPE + 2)

Black: Recovery (Base pace RPE - 1)

Light Gray: Cool-down* (RPE 4-5)

*Optional: Continue praying the 2nd Rosary during the cool-down period

End with the Hail Holy Queen, even if you don't finish a 2nd Rosary

Resume your base pace RPE during the recovery, when, or if you are able.

Continue the 6th interval through the Our Father and 1st mystery announcement of the 2nd Rosary.
(See arrow)

You will skip the other prayers on the pendant chain of the 2nd Rosary

Workout 2 – Recovery (30 minutes total time):

Focus: These active recovery workouts offer an excellent opportunity to practice meditation and reflect on your readings for this level.

Workout: After the **Throne Level Warm-up**, increase intensity to your recovery pace (base pace RPE minus one) as you pray the Rosary during a 30-minute workout. For some exercisers, the warm-up pace and the recovery pace are essentially the same. When you finish the Rosary, transition to the **Throne Level Cool-down**.

Journal entry: Log your workout in your journal.

Workout 3 – Long Intervals (30 minutes total time):

Focus: Today you'll add a 4th long interval, incorporating the shorter recovery times between intervals. Refer to Week 1, Workout 3 above to review the detailed instructions. A graphic depiction follows the instructions below.

Workout: After the **Throne Level Warm-up**, increase intensity to your base pace (RPE of 5-6) and begin praying the Rosary.

The first long interval begins with the 2nd decade of Hail Mary's. The interval pace is base pace RPE + 1. Recover from the Glory Be to the Our Father.

Repeat this long interval, short recovery pattern during the 3rd, 4th and 5th decades. The recovery period for the 5th decade is slightly different as you'll recover during the Glory Be, Fatima Prayer and Hail Holy Queen and then transition to the **Throne Level Cool-down**. You may want to increase the duration of your cool-down today.

<u>Journal entry</u>: Log the workout in your journal. Be sure to add notes about any revelations or thoughts you experienced during your Rosary meditation.

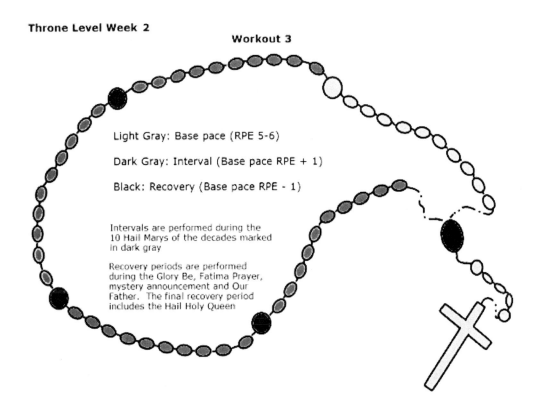

Throne Level Week 2

Workout 3

Light Gray: Base pace (RPE 5-6)

Dark Gray: Interval (Base pace RPE + 1)

Black: Recovery (Base pace RPE - 1)

Intervals are performed during the 10 Hail Marys of the decades marked in dark gray

Recovery periods are performed during the Glory Be, Fatima Prayer, mystery announcement and Our Father. The final recovery period includes the Hail Holy Queen

Workout 4 - Recovery (30 minutes total):

<u>Workout</u>: Following the **Throne Level Warm-up**, increase intensity to your recovery pace (base pace RPE minus one), and include **unstructured time** ideas during a 30-minute recovery workout. Transition to the **Throne Level Cool-down** during the last 5 minutes.

<u>Journal entry</u>: Log your workout in your journal.

Spiritual Component: Continue reading the source you've chosen.

Note: This week we begin the Advanced Workout cycle: a short interval workout followed by a long interval workout, then a recovery day. If you become overly sore or fatigued or experience overtraining symptoms, then modify the workouts. Feel free to add an extra recovery workout any time in the program.

Workout 1 – Short Intervals (40-50 minutes total time):

Focus: Today you'll increase the number of short intervals to nine or ten total.

Workout: After the **Throne Level Warm-up**, increase intensity to your base pace (RPE of 5-6), and pray the first Rosary while completing five short intervals. Continue with the 6th, 7th, 8th and 9th intervals, according to the instructions for Week 2, Workout 1.

The 10th interval begins with the Glory Be at the end of the fourth decade of the second Rosary and ends with the Our Father. Recover during the rest of the Rosary, then transition to the **Throne Level Cool-down**.

Journal entry: Log the workout in your journal.

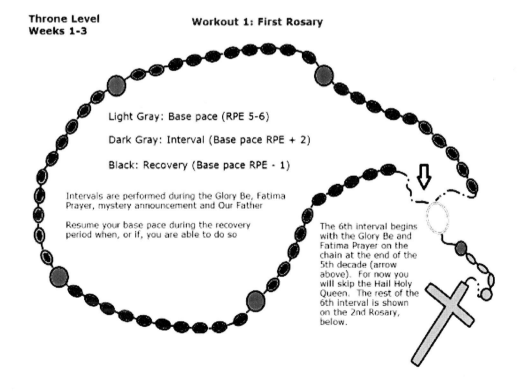

Throne Level
Weeks 1-3

Workout 1: First Rosary

Light Gray: Base pace (RPE 5-6)

Dark Gray: Interval (Base pace RPE + 2)

Black: Recovery (Base pace RPE - 1)

Intervals are performed during the Glory Be, Fatima Prayer, mystery announcement and Our Father

Resume your base pace during the recovery period when, or if, you are able to do so

The 6th interval begins with the Glory Be and Fatima Prayer on the chain at the end of the 5th decade (arrow above). For now you will skip the Hail Holy Queen. The rest of the 6th interval is shown on the 2nd Rosary, below.

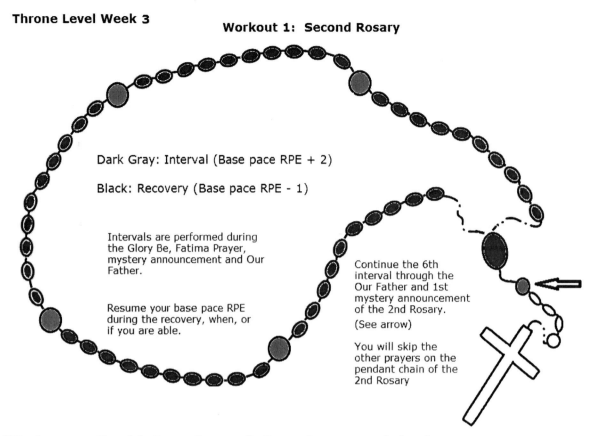

Throne Level Week 3

Workout 1: Second Rosary

Dark Gray: Interval (Base pace RPE + 2)

Black: Recovery (Base pace RPE - 1)

Intervals are performed during the Glory Be, Fatima Prayer, mystery announcement and Our Father.

Resume your base pace RPE during the recovery, when, or if you are able.

Continue the 6th interval through the Our Father and 1st mystery announcement of the 2nd Rosary.
(See arrow)

You will skip the other prayers on the pendant chain of the 2nd Rosary

Workout 2 – Double Long Intervals (30 minutes total time):

Focus: Today you'll try a new type of interval: double long intervals. The double long interval increases the duration by continuing the increased pace through two full decades. The goal is to complete two double long intervals. A graphic of the workout follows the instructions below.

Continue to master the challenge of Rosary meditation during a tough interval workout. Train your mind to focus on the mysteries rather than the physical discomfort.

Note: Extend the warm-up time a bit today as the intervals begin fairly early in the workout.

Workout: After the **Throne Level Warm-up**, increase intensity to your base pace (RPE of 5-6) and begin praying the Rosary. Pray all the pendant chain prayers.

The **first double long interval** will begin with the 1st decade of Hail Mary's. Increase your pace slightly to base pace RPE + 1. Your goal is to maintain the interval pace through the 10 Hail Mary's of the 1st decade, Glory Be, Fatima Prayer, 2nd mystery announcement, Our Father and 10 Hail Mary's of the 2nd decade. Whew! The recovery period begins with the Glory Be, continues through the rest of the 3rd decade and ends with the Our Father at the beginning of the 4th decade. Resume your base pace RPE when, or if, you are able.

The **second double long interval** begins with the 4th decade of Hail Mary's and continues through the Glory Be, Fatima Prayer, 5th mystery announcement, Our Father and 10 Hail Mary's of the 5th decade. Recover during the Glory Be, Fatima Prayer and Hail Holy Queen and transition to the **Throne Level Cool-down**. Extend your cool-down period today.

Journal entry: Log your workout in your journal.

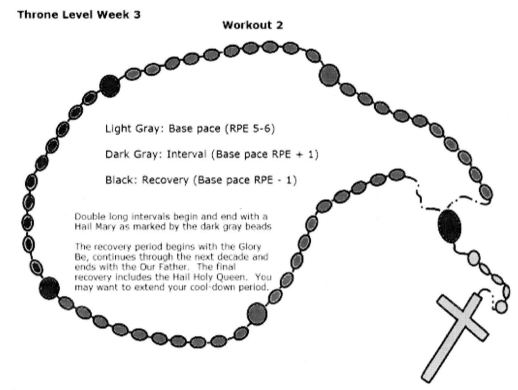

Throne Level Week 3

Workout 2

Light Gray: Base pace (RPE 5-6)

Dark Gray: Interval (Base pace RPE + 1)

Black: Recovery (Base pace RPE - 1)

Double long intervals begin and end with a Hail Mary as marked by the dark gray beads

The recovery period begins with the Glory Be, continues through the next decade and ends with the Our Father. The final recovery includes the Hail Holy Queen. You may want to extend your cool-down period.

Workout 3 – Recovery (30 minutes):

Focus: You really earned this recovery workout! Enjoy the relaxing effect of exercise at an easy pace and experience how your muscles loosen up as your body works to remove the accumulated exercise by-products. A long post-workout stretching session helps with this process.

Workout: After the **Throne Level Warm-up**, increase intensity to your recovery pace (base pace RPE minus one) and pray the Rosary during a 30-minute workout. When you finish the Rosary, transition to the **Throne Level Cool-down**.

Journal entry: Log your workout in your journal.

Workout 4 – Base Pace Training (30 minutes)

Workout: Following the **Throne Level Warm-up**, increase intensity to your base pace (RPE 5-6), and include **unstructured time** ideas during a 30-minute recovery workout. Transition to the **Throne Level Cool-down** during the last 5 minutes.

Journal entry: Log your workout in your journal.

"Give me an army saying the Rosary and I will conquer the world." -Pope Pius IX

Throne Level Week 4 (Recovery Week)

Spiritual Component: Finish reading the source you've chosen.

Workout 1 – Short Intervals (20-30 minutes total time):

Focus: Since this is a recovery week, decrease the number of intervals. A total of 4-5 is sufficient. Decrease the workout duration to 20-30 minutes.

Workout: Following the **Throne Level Warm-up**, increase intensity to your base pace (RPE of 5-6), and pray the Rosary while completing 4-5 short intervals. When you finish the Rosary, transition to the **Throne Level Cool-down**.

Journal entry: Log your workout in your journal.

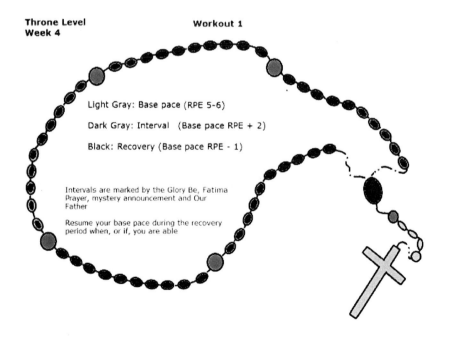

Throne Level
Week 4

Workout 1

Light Gray: Base pace (RPE 5-6)

Dark Gray: Interval (Base pace RPE + 2)

Black: Recovery (Base pace RPE - 1)

Intervals are marked by the Glory Be, Fatima Prayer, mystery announcement and Our Father

Resume your base pace during the recovery period when, or if, you are able

Workout 2 – Recovery (30 minutes total time):

Focus: During the cool-down, think of a good deed that you can do later today. Remember that you're trying to <u>live</u> the Gospels!

Workout: After the **Throne Level Warm-up**, increase intensity to your recovery pace (base pace RPE minus one) as you pray the Rosary during a 30-minute workout. When you finish the Rosary, transition to the **Throne Level Cool-down**.

Journal entry: Log your workout in your journal.

Workout 3 – Long Intervals (30 minutes total time):

Focus: Today is a long-interval workout day. Since this is a recovery week, decrease the length of the long interval to just one decade.

Workout: After the **Throne Level Warm-up**, increase intensity to your base pace (RPE of 5-6), and begin praying the Rosary. The long interval will begin with the 2nd decade of Hail Mary's. Increase your pace slightly to base pace RPE + 1, and maintain the interval pace as you pray the 10 Hail Mary's. The recovery period begins with the Glory Be at the end of the 2nd decade and continues through the rest of the 3rd decade. Resume your base pace when you can, and continue praying the rest of the Rosary. Transition to the **Throne Level Cool-down** when you finish the Rosary.

Journal entry: Log your workout in your journal.

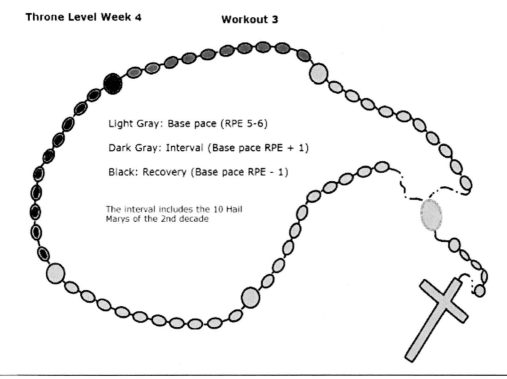

Throne Level Week 4   Workout 3

Light Gray: Base pace (RPE 5-6)

Dark Gray: Interval (Base pace RPE + 1)

Black: Recovery (Base pace RPE - 1)

The interval includes the 10 Hail
Marys of the 2nd decade

Workout 4 – Recovery (30 minutes):

Focus: For a change of pace, invite a friend or family member to accompany you during your workout. Perhaps you might discuss the Rosary mysteries, the Bible or the book you're reading for this level. If you can't find a willing exercise partner, talk to your guardian angel as you would with a friend. Listen for your angel's guidance today.

Workout: After the **Throne Level Warm-up**, exercise at recovery pace (base pace RPE minus one), and use **unstructured time** ideas during a 30-minute recovery workout. Transition to the **Throne Level Cool-down** during the last 5 minutes.

Journal entry: Log your workout in your journal.

Congratulations on completing the Throne Level of The Rosary Workout™!

Take care of your body. It's the only place you have to live. - Jim Rohn

Throne Level Graduation Requirements

You are ready to move on to the Cherubim Level if you have met the following conditions:

1. You have exercised 4 days each week for 4 continuous weeks.
2. You are able to complete 10 short intervals.
3. You can complete two double long intervals: 2 decades of the Rosary at an interval pace of base pace RPE + 1
4. You have no symptoms of overtraining.
5. You have expanded your study of the Rosary by reading the Bible, papal documents, writings of the saints, or other sources.
6a. If you have not met the conditions above, consider extra study and/or workouts before you progress to the Cherubim Level. If intervals are too challenging, make sure that you're not trying to push yourself past your limits. Remember that the workout descriptions are a goal, not a requirement. Take as much time as you need to finish the Throne Level.
6b. If you can't seem to find the time to fit in the spiritual exercises, then take a good look at your schedule. Perhaps you can substitute a short Bible study for time spent surfing the web. Turn off the TV and read a chapter from a book on the Rosary or about a saint you're studying. Look for other little chunks of time that you can use to improve your spiritual fitness.
7. Reward yourself for reaching your goal.
8. Don't forget to pray to the Choir of Thrones (and any saints to whom you prayed for intercession) to thank them for their assistance in helping you complete this level.

Throne Level Completion Assignments:

For the Soul: Don't forget to go to Confession! Your assignment for this month is to continue expanding your study of the Rosary. Go back to the beginning of the Throne Level and re-read the list of resources to find another one that interests you. An alternative is to view some of the programs on EWTN or buy or rent videos or DVDs about the lives of the saints, Catholic history, and other interesting topics. Check out Pius Media for a list of titles for rent: **www.piusmedia.com**

For the Body: Go to your local library or bookstore and look through the cookbook section. Choose a health-themed cookbook that appeals to you and try at least one new recipe. Or, buy a magazine such as Cooking Light, Eating Well, etc. and try at least one new recipe. Many magazines have associated websites where recipes are published and reviewed by users.

Cherubim Level Workouts: Second Advanced Level (4 weeks)

Prayer to the **Choir of Cherubim:**

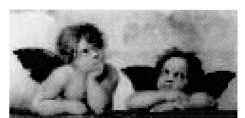

By the intercession of St. Michael and the celestial Choir of Cherubim may the Lord grant us the grace to leave the ways of sin and run in the paths of Christian perfection. Amen

-From the Chaplet of St. Michael the Archangel

Pray to the Cherubim Choir and your own guardian angel for help in completing this level.

Cherubim Level Summary and Goals:

The Cherubim Level workouts continue to build intensity by slowly increasing the number of short intervals and the duration of long intervals. You'll also increase the workout frequency to five days a week. A fun "Rosary Race" is introduced in Week 3.

To continue your progress in Mary's School of the Rosary, I will challenge you to practice the virtues embedded in each of the 20 mysteries.

Goals:

1. Increase frequency to 5 days per week.

Note: If you cannot exercise more than three or four times a week, you can still complete the Cherubim Level. Accomplish the workouts in order, but only do three (or four) workouts each week. Obviously, this will take more than 4 weeks, and the peak and recovery weeks won't line up. Modify the program as needed to fit your schedule. You may also need to increase the duration of some of the Cherubim Level workouts to 40-60+ minutes so that you maintain the fitness level you reached during the previous levels. Refer to your journal to help you plan the workouts. Specific instructions are not included for these modifications.

2. Increase the duration of long intervals

3. Apply the advanced workout cycle: A day of short interval workouts followed by a day of longer intervals, followed by a recovery day.

4. Study the virtues associated with each of the twenty mysteries of the Rosary

By the end of the Cherubim Level you will be able to:

1. Pray the Rosary during exercise 5 days each week

2. Complete a Rosary Race

3. Understand the virtues associated with each mystery of the Rosary

Spiritual Component for the Cherubim Level:

You will study the virtues associated with each mystery and learn to apply them in your own life. The Catechism of the Catholic Church and Pope John Paul II's *Rosary of the Virgin Mary* are excellent resources to learn more about the virtues portrayed in the Rosary.

Exercise Components for the Cherubim Level:

Frequency: 5 days per week

Duration: 30 - 60 minutes each workout

Intensity:

Warm-up and Cool-down: Moderate to Somewhat Hard (4-5 on RPE scale)

Base pace: Somewhat Hard to Very Hard (5-7 on RPE scale)

Short intervals: Base pace RPE + 2

Long intervals: Base pace RPE + 1

Recovery: Base pace RPE minus 1

Note: Adjust the RPE suggestions above, based on your current fitness level

Mode: Any type of rhythmic aerobic exercise

Cherubim Level Warm-up: The Cherubim Level warm-up is the same throughout all the workouts in this level and is therefore listed only once. As you begin the physical portion of the warm-up, you should also "warm-up" spiritually. Begin exercise at an RPE of 4-5 while you say a short prayer to the Holy Spirit, your patron saint or the Blessed Mother asking for help in applying the virtues of each mystery to your own life. Decide on a Rosary intention based on your own needs or those of others. The warm-up should last at least 5 minutes and perhaps longer if indicated in the workout instructions. You are ready to begin your workout with the opening prayer of the Rosary, The Apostles' Creed.

Cherubim Level Cool-down: The Cherubim Level cool-down is also the same throughout all the workouts in this level. Slow your pace to an RPE of 4-5 for at least 5 minutes. Use this time to reflect on the mysteries, think of a good deed you can do today, or enjoy your surroundings and the great feeling of accomplishment in finishing your workout.

Stretch: If time allows after your workout, take a few minutes to stretch the major muscle groups you worked during exercise. If you don't have time to stretch, try to fit in a stretching session later in the day or at least 2-3 times each week.

Cherubim Level Week 1

Spiritual Component: Study the virtue for each mystery and reflect on how you can apply it to your own life. This week, you'll focus on the virtues of the Joyful Mysteries.

Workout 1 – Short Intervals (40-50 minutes total time):

Focus: Today your goal is to complete ten short intervals as you pray two Rosaries. Recall that a short interval is defined as an increased pace (base pace RPE + 2) during the Glory Be, Fatima Prayer, mystery announcement and Our Father at the beginning of a given decade. The recovery period is marked by the following 10 Hail Mary's. The workout duration will be approximately 40-50 minutes. A graphic depiction of the workout follows the detailed instructions below.

Reflect on the Joyful Mysteries today, especially the first Joyful Mystery, The Annunciation and its associated virtue, humility. How can you become a more humble person? How often do you put others' needs before your own?

Note: You can still accomplish 10 intervals without praying a second Rosary. Use a watch or other timing device to determine the duration of each interval and recovery period as you complete the first five intervals while praying the first Rosary. During the 6th-10th intervals, delete the references to the second Rosary and use timing instead. As a guide, the short intervals usually last about 45-60 seconds to complete. The recovery period (10 Hail Mary's) lasts about 2 minutes.

Workout: After **Cherubim Level Warm-up** increase intensity to your base pace (RPE of 5-7), and pray the Rosary while completing ten short intervals. Interval pace is base pace RPE + 2. The first interval is marked on the pendant chain and begins with the Glory Be after the 3 Hail Mary's and continues through the Our Father. Recover during the first 10 Hail Mary's on the circular chain. Recovery pace is base pace RPE minus 1.

Continue this interval and recovery pattern with the 2nd, 3rd, 4th and 5th decades.

During the sixth interval, you will begin a second Rosary. This interval is the same length of time as previous intervals, but the marking of the prayers on the Rosary is slightly different because you are transitioning to the second Rosary.

The interval begins with the Glory Be and Fatima Prayer at the end of the 5th decade (you will skip the Hail Holy Queen, marked by the medal in the center of the Rosary, for now). Continue the interval pace as you announce the first mystery of a new set of mysteries (see note below) and the Our Father, which are marked by the last bead on the pendant chain.

Note: You will not pray the other prayers on the pendant chain (Apostles' Creed and three Hail Mary's) for this second Rosary. The second set of mysteries is simply a different set than those you meditated upon during the first Rosary. For example, if you prayed the first Rosary while meditating on the Joyful Mysteries, then you will pray the second Rosary while meditating on a the Luminous, Sorrowful or Glorious, your choice). Of course, you can always repeat the same set of mysteries, especially if you were distracted or had trouble meditating during the first Rosary.

Recover during the 10 Hail Mary's of the first new mystery. Recovery RPE is base pace RPE minus one. (Although this is really your 6th decade, it is marked by the first 10 Hail Mary's after the center medal.) Resume your base pace RPE when you are able.

The 7th, 8th, and 9th intervals follow the same pattern as the first Rosary. The 10th interval begins with the Glory Be at the end of the fourth decade of the second Rosary and ends with the Our Father. Recover during the rest of the Rosary, then transition to the **Cherubim Level Cool-down**.

Journal entry: Log your workout in your journal.

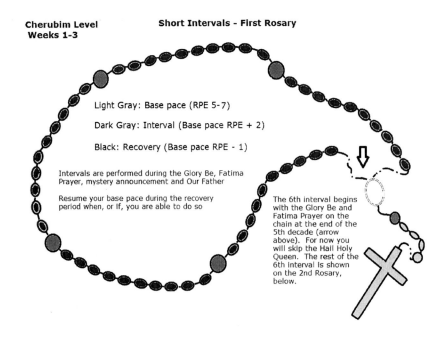

Cherubim Level
Weeks 1-3

Short Intervals - First Rosary

Light Gray: Base pace (RPE 5-7)

Dark Gray: Interval (Base pace RPE + 2)

Black: Recovery (Base pace RPE - 1)

Intervals are performed during the Glory Be, Fatima Prayer, mystery announcement and Our Father

Resume your base pace during the recovery period when, or if, you are able to do so

The 6th interval begins with the Glory Be and Fatima Prayer on the chain at the end of the 5th decade (arrow above). For now you will skip the Hail Holy Queen. The rest of the 6th interval is shown on the 2nd Rosary, below.

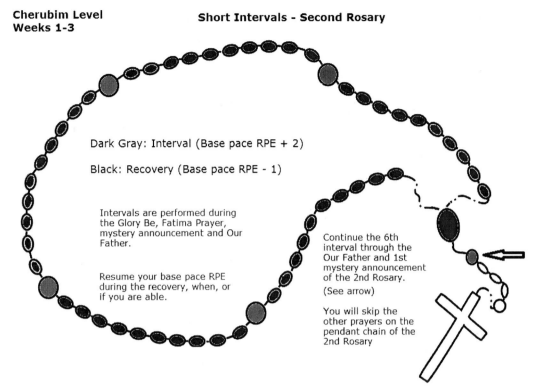

Cherubim Level Weeks 1-3

Short Intervals - Second Rosary

Dark Gray: Interval (Base pace RPE + 2)

Black: Recovery (Base pace RPE - 1)

Intervals are performed during the Glory Be, Fatima Prayer, mystery announcement and Our Father.

Resume your base pace RPE during the recovery, when, or if you are able.

Continue the 6th interval through the Our Father and 1st mystery announcement of the 2nd Rosary.

(See arrow)

You will skip the other prayers on the pendant chain of the 2nd Rosary

<u>Note:</u> Use these two graphics for all short interval workouts in Weeks 1-3

Workout 2 – Double Long Intervals (30 minutes total time):

<u>Note:</u> From now on, you will incorporate the Advanced Workout cycle: A day of short interval workouts followed by a day of longer intervals, followed by a recovery day. If you are overly sore or fatigued from yesterday's workout or experience overtraining symptoms, then modify the plan as needed.

<u>Focus:</u> Today you will continue to increase intensity by decreasing the recovery period between the double long intervals. Recall that a double long interval is defined as maintaining an interval pace (base pace RPE + 1) for two continuous decades of the Rosary. Refer to your journal notes from the Throne Level if needed. You may want to extend your warm-up time a bit today as the intervals begin fairly early in the workout.

Reflect on the Joyful Mysteries today, especially the second Joyful Mystery, The Visitation and its associated virtue, charity and love of neighbor. How can you be charitable to your neighbor today?

<u>Workout:</u> After the **Cherubim Level Warm-up**, increase intensity to your base pace (RPE of 5-7) and begin praying the Rosary. Pray all the pendant chain prayers.

The **first double long interval** begins with the 1st decade of ten Hail Mary's and ends with the 10th Hail Mary of the 2nd decade. The recovery period is very short—it begins with the Glory Be and continues through the Our Father. The interval pace is base pace RPE + 1, and recovery pace is base pace RPE minus one.

The **second double long interval** begins with the 3rd decade of ten Hail Mary's and ends with the 10th Hail Mary of the 4th decade. Recover during the rest of the Rosary, then transition to the **Cherubim Level Cool-down**.

<u>**Journal entry**</u>: Log your workout in your journal.

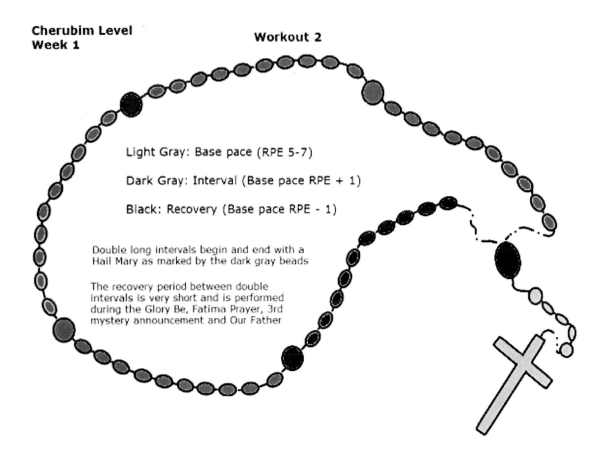

Cherubim Level
Week 1

Workout 2

Light Gray: Base pace (RPE 5-7)

Dark Gray: Interval (Base pace RPE + 1)

Black: Recovery (Base pace RPE - 1)

Double long intervals begin and end with a Hail Mary as marked by the dark gray beads

The recovery period between double intervals is very short and is performed during the Glory Be, Fatima Prayer, 3rd mystery announcement and Our Father

Workout 3 – Recovery (30-45 minutes):

<u>**Focus:**</u> This workout is most effective when done the day after an interval workout. Do not skip these recovery workouts as adaptation occurs during recovery and not during the overload (interval workouts). A graphic of this workout is depicted in the Throne Level.

Reflect on the third Joyful Mystery, The Nativity, and its associated virtue, poverty. Can you give up something today that you'd like to buy and give the money to the poor? Can you live a more simple life and detach yourself from material possessions?

Workout: After the **Cherubim Level Warm-up**, increase intensity to your recovery pace (base pace RPE minus one), and include suggestions for **unstructured time** during a 30-45 minute workout. If you choose not to pray the Rosary, then spend a few minutes reflecting on The Nativity and the virtue of poverty. Transition to the **Cherubim Level Cool-down** during the last 5 minutes of the workout.

Journal entry: Log your workout in your journal.

Workout 4 – Short Intervals (40-50 minutes)

Focus: Reflect on the Joyful Mysteries today, especially the fourth Joyful Mystery, The Presentation, and its associated virtue, obedience. Do you always obey the law and other types of authority? What about the Ten Commandments and the teachings of the Catholic Church?

Workout: After the **Cherubim Level Warm-up**, increase intensity to your base pace (RPE of 5-7) and complete 10 short intervals. You can accomplish the intervals while praying two Rosaries, or praying one Rosary and using timing for the last five intervals or simply use timing for all the intervals and include **unstructured time** ideas during recovery periods. If you choose not to pray the Rosary, then spend some time reflecting on The Presentation and the virtue of obedience. Transition to the **Cherubim Level Cool-down** during the last 5 minutes of the workout.

Journal entry: Log your workout in your journal. Jot down any timing references you used to help you in planning future interval workouts.

Workout 5 – Triple Long Interval (30 minutes total time):

Focus: Today your goal is to complete a triple long interval l-- maintaining an interval pace for three continuous decades of the Rosary.

Reflect on the Joyful Mysteries today, especially the fifth Joyful Mystery, The Finding of the Child Jesus in the Temple and its associated virtue, joy in finding Jesus. Do you seek Jesus' presence in your life? Do you listen for His voice in prayer?

Workout: After the **Cherubim Level Warm-up**, increase intensity to your base pace (RPE of 5-7) and begin praying the Rosary.

The **triple long interval** begins with the 2nd decade of ten Hail Mary's. Increase your pace slightly to base pace RPE + 1 and maintain the interval pace through three continuous decades (through the 10th Hail Mary of the 4th decade, about 8-10 minutes). The recovery period is the rest of the Rosary at a pace of base pace RPE minus one. Transition to the **Cherubim Level Cool-down** when you finish the Rosary.

Optional: Add extra time at your base pace RPE, using suggestions for **unstructured time**.

Journal entry: Log your workout in your journal.

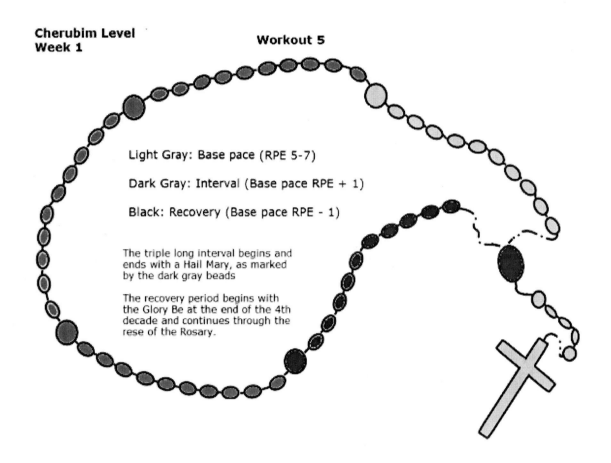

Cherubim Level Week 1

Workout 5

Light Gray: Base pace (RPE 5-7)

Dark Gray: Interval (Base pace RPE + 1)

Black: Recovery (Base pace RPE - 1)

The triple long interval begins and ends with a Hail Mary, as marked by the dark gray beads

The recovery period begins with the Glory Be at the end of the 4th decade and continues through the rese of the Rosary.

"St. Dominic knew well that, while on the one hand Mary is all powerful with her divine Son, who grants all graces to mankind through her, on the other hand, she is by nature so good and so merciful that, inclined to aid spontaneously those who suffer, she is absolutely incapable of refusing her help to those who invoke her. The Church is in the habit of greeting the Virgin as 'Mother of Grace' and 'Mother of Mercy,' and so she has always shown herself, especially when we have recourse to her by means of the Holy Rosary." -Pope Benedict XV

<u>Spiritual Component</u>: Study the virtue for each mystery and reflect on how you can apply it to your own life. This week, you'll focus on the virtues of the Luminous Mysteries.

Workout 1 – Recovery (30-45 minutes total time):

<u>Focus:</u> Reflect on the Luminous Mysteries today, especially the first Luminous Mystery, The Baptism of Jesus and its associated virtue, fidelity to our baptismal promises. Are you faithful to the promises of Baptism? Do you know what they are?

<u>Workout:</u> After the **Cherubim Level Warm-up**, increase intensity to your recovery pace (base pace RPE minus one), and include suggestions for **unstructured time** during a 30-45 minute workout. If you choose not to pray the Rosary today, spend some time reflecting on The Baptism of Jesus and the virtue of faithfulness to your baptismal promises. Transition to the **Cherubim Level Cool-down** during the last 5 minutes of the workout.

<u>Journal entry</u>: Log your workout in your journal.

Workout 2 – Short Intervals (40-50 minutes total time):

<u>Focus:</u> Reflect on the Luminous Mysteries today, especially the second Luminous Mystery, The Wedding Feast at Cana and its associated virtue, faith in Mary's intercession and maternal care. Do you ask for Mary's assistance and guidance in becoming more like Christ? Do you follow the example she set?

<u>Workout:</u> After the **Cherubim Level Warm-up**, increase intensity to your base pace (RPE of 5-7) and complete 10 short intervals. You can accomplish the intervals while praying two Rosaries, or praying one Rosary and using timing for the last five intervals or simply use timing for all the intervals and include **unstructured time** ideas during recovery periods. If you choose not to pray the Rosary, spend some time reflecting on The Wedding Feast at Cana and the virtue of faith in Mary's intercession and maternal care. Transition to the **Cherubim Level Cool-down** during the last 5 minutes of the workout.

<u>Journal entry</u>: Log your workout in your journal.

Workout 3 – Quadruple Long Interval (30 minutes total time):

<u>Focus:</u> Today your goal is to complete a quadruple long interval -- maintaining an interval pace (base pace RPE + 1) for four continuous decades of the Rosary.

Reflect on the Luminous Mysteries today, especially the third Luminous Mystery, The Proclamation of the Kingdom and its associated virtue, conversion of heart. Have you turned from sin and vowed to live a virtuous life? Do you model your life on the Beatitudes?

Workout: After the **Cherubim Level Warm-up**, increase intensity to your base pace (RPE of 5-7) and begin praying the Rosary. You might want to warm up longer than usual as the interval begins fairly early in the workout.

The **quadruple long interval** begins with the 1st decade of ten Hail Mary's. Increase your pace slightly to base pace RPE + 1 and maintain the interval pace through four continuous decades (through the 10th Hail Mary of the 4th decade, about 13-15 minutes). The recovery period is the rest of the Rosary at a pace of base pace RPE minus one. Transition to the **Cherubim Level Cool-down** when you finish the Rosary.

Optional: Add additional time at your base pace RPE, and include suggestions for **unstructured time**.

Journal entry: Log your workout in your journal. Be sure to add notes about any revelations or thoughts you experienced during your Rosary meditation.

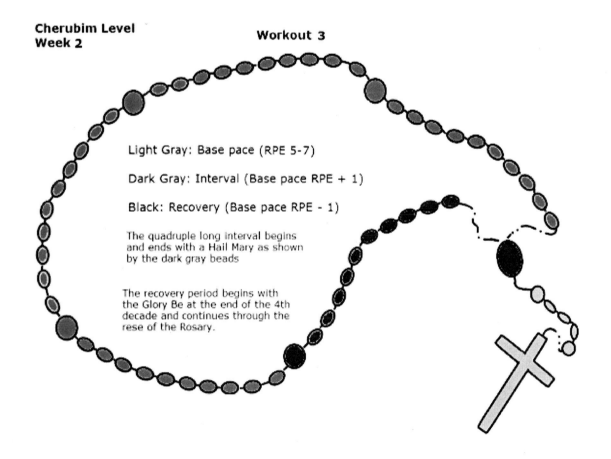

**Cherubim Level
Week 2**

Workout 3

Light Gray: Base pace (RPE 5-7)

Dark Gray: Interval (Base pace RPE + 1)

Black: Recovery (Base pace RPE - 1)

The quadruple long interval begins
and ends with a Hail Mary as shown
by the dark gray beads

The recovery period begins with
the Glory Be at the end of the 4th
decade and continues through the
rese of the Rosary.

Workout 4 – Recovery (30-45 minutes):

Focus: Reflect on the Luminous Mysteries today, especially the fourth Luminous Mystery, The Transfiguration and its associated virtue, desire to become a new person in Christ. Have you changed your life to become more like Christ? Do you look for the presence of Jesus in others?

Workout: After the **Cherubim Level Warm-up**, increase intensity to your recovery pace (base pace RPE minus one), and include suggestions for **unstructured time** during a 30-45 minute workout. If you choose not to pray the Rosary today, then spend some time reflecting on The Transfiguration and the virtue of desiring to become a new person in Christ. Transition to the **Cherubim Level Cool-down** during the last 5 minutes of the workout.

Journal entry: Log your workout in your journal.

Workout 5 – Short Intervals (40-50 minutes):

Focus: Reflect on the Luminous Mysteries today, especially the fifth Luminous Mystery, The Institution of the Eucharist and its associated virtue, love of the Eucharist and active participation at Mass. Do you actively participate in Mass? Are you truly prepared to receive Jesus in the Eucharist?

Workout: After the **Cherubim Level Warm-up**, increase intensity to your base pace (RPE of 5-7) and complete 10 short intervals. You can accomplish the intervals while praying two Rosaries, or praying one Rosary and using timing for the last five intervals or simply use timing for all the intervals and include **unstructured time** ideas during recovery periods. If you choose not to pray the Rosary today, then spend some time reflecting on The Institution of the Eucharist and the virtue of active participation in Mass and readiness to receive Jesus in the Eucharist. Transition to the **Cherubim Level Cool-down** during the last 5 minutes of the workout.

Journal entry: Log your workout in your journal.

"Virtue is like health: the harmony of the whole man." - Thomas Carlyle

Cherubim Level Week 3 (Peak Week)

Spiritual Component: Study the virtue for each mystery and reflect on how you can apply it to your own life. This week, you'll focus on the virtues of the Sorrowful Mysteries.

Workout 1 – Base Pace Training (30-40 minutes total time):

Focus: This workout breaks up the advanced workout cycle you've been using for the last few weeks, but it's designed to prepare you for a fun challenge later this week. Today you'll work on base pace training — maintaining a constant pace during a 30-40 minute workout.

Use the combined rhythm of the constant pace and the repeated Rosary prayers to clear your mind for deeper meditative prayer.

Reflect on the Sorrowful Mysteries today, especially the first Sorrowful Mystery, The Agony in the Garden and its associated virtue, repentance and true sorrow for sin. Have you gone to Confession recently? Are there any sinful practices in your life that you can eliminate?

Workout: After the **Cherubim Level Warm-up**, increase intensity to your base pace (RPE of 5-7), and pray the Rosary during a 30-40 minute workout. Since you'll likely finish the Rosary before the recommended duration, include suggestions for **unstructured time** during the additional time. Transition to the **Cherubim Level Cool-down** during the last 5 minutes of the workout.

Journal entry: Log your workout in your journal.

Workout 2 – Recovery (20-30 minutes):

Focus: This is a short and easy workout before your next challenge — a Rosary Race.

Reflect on the Sorrowful Mysteries today, especially the second Sorrowful Mystery, The Scourging at the Pillar and its associated virtue, modesty and purity along with self-denial. Do you dress modestly? Do you indulge in impure thoughts or practices? Is there some comfort or luxury that you can deny yourself to practice self-control?

Workout: Following the **Cherubim Level Warm-up,** increase intensity to your recovery pace (base pace RPE minus one), and include suggestions for **unstructured time** during a 20-30 minute workout. If you choose not to pray the Rosary today, then spend some time reflecting on The Scourging at the Pillar and the virtues of modesty, purity and self-denial. Transition to the **Cherubim Level Cool-down** during the last 5 minutes of the workout.

Journal entry: Log your workout in your journal.

Workout 3 – Rosary Race (30 minutes total time):

Focus: Today's workout is a fun challenge: A Rosary Race! Choose a course that will take about 20 minutes to complete. The race course will depend on your usual mode of exercise. If you walk or run, use the track at your local high school or community college (call first to be sure it's okay), or a jogging/biking path. If you bike, find a bike path or a long, straight road with minimal traffic. If you swim, try an Olympic pool or an open water swim in a lake or river (always use a safety observer!).

If weather is an issue, find an indoor track or walk or run in a shopping mall before it opens to the public (most malls are open early for "Mall Walkers"). Another option is to use a treadmill or stationary bike in a gym or city recreation center. Many gyms will sell a one-day pass if you don't have a membership.

The goal of the Rosary Race is to cover as much distance as possible while praying the Rosary. If you're outside, use landmarks to determine your start and finish points. If you're in a gym, reset the time and distance display after the warm-up when you're ready to start the race.

Repeat the Rosary Race, using the same course or cardio equipment, once a month or so to measure improvement.

Reflect on the Sorrowful Mysteries today, especially the third Sorrowful Mystery, The Crowning of Thorns and its associated virtue, love of your enemies and moral courage. Do you pray for your enemies? Do you forgive and <u>forget</u>? Do you have the moral courage to do what is right, even when it's difficult? Do you look for the presence of Jesus in people whom you dislike?

<u>Workout:</u> Complete the **Cherubim Level Warm-up**. It's a good idea to extend the warm-up time a few minutes in preparation for the race. Start the race as you begin the Apostles' Creed. Your RPE for the race should be about base pace RPE +1. Continue at this race pace until you've prayed an entire Rosary. If you get tired during the race, slow your pace for a minute or two, then try to resume your race pace after you've caught your breath. When you finish the Rosary, transition to the **Cherubim Level Cool-down**.

<u>Journal entry</u>: Log your workout in your journal. Include as many details about your Rosary Race as possible — RPE, distance covered (or note landmarks), weather, how you felt during and after the race, etc.

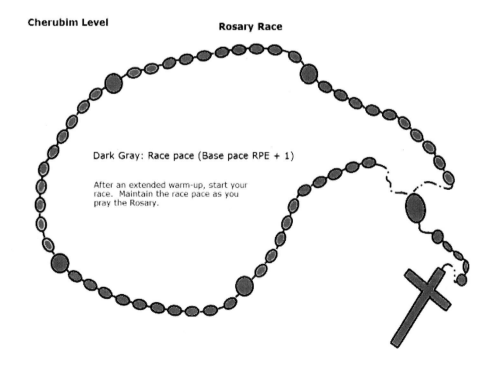

Cherubim Level　　　　**Rosary Race**

Dark Gray: Race pace (Base pace RPE + 1)

After an extended warm-up, start your race. Maintain the race pace as you pray the Rosary.

Workout 4 – Recovery (30-45 minutes total time):

Focus: This workout is designed to be easy and serves as an active recovery following your Rosary Race. It's most effective when done the day after the race.

Reflect on the Sorrowful Mysteries today, especially the fourth Sorrowful Mystery, The Carrying of the Cross and its associated virtue, patience in suffering and fortitude. Do you complain or try to place blame when life doesn't go your way, or do you quietly bear your crosses? Do you find strength through prayer during trials and trust in God's plan for you?

Workout: Following the **Cherubim Level Warm-up** increase intensity to your recovery pace (base pace RPE minus one), and include suggestions for **unstructured time** during a 20-30 minute workout. If you choose not to pray the Rosary today, then spend some time reflecting on The Carrying of the Cross and the virtues of patience in suffering and fortitude. Transition to the **Cherubim Level Cool-down** during the last 5 minutes of the workout.

Journal entry: Log your workout in your journal.

Workout 5 – Short Intervals (40-50 minutest total time):

Focus: Reflect on the Sorrowful Mysteries today, especially the fifth Sorrowful Mystery, The Crucifixion and its associated virtue, perseverance and mercy. Do you persevere in your faith? Do you show mercy, even when you think it's not deserved?

Workout: After the **Cherubim Level Warm-up**, increase intensity to your base pace (RPE of 5-7) and complete 10 short intervals. You can accomplish the intervals while praying two Rosaries, or praying one Rosary and using timing for the last five intervals or simply use timing for all the intervals and include **unstructured time** ideas during recovery periods. If you choose not to pray the Rosary today, then spend some time reflecting on The Crucifixion and the virtues of perseverance and mercy.

Journal entry: Log your workout in your journal.

"True enjoyment comes from activity of the mind and exercise of the body; the two are united." - Alexander von Humboldt

---

Cherubim Level Week 4 (Recovery Week)

<u>Spiritual Component</u>: Study the virtue for each mystery and reflect on how you can apply it to your own life. This week, you'll focus on the virtues of the Glorious Mysteries.

Workout 1 – Long Intervals (30 minutes total time):

Focus: Since this is a recovery week, this long interval workout is less challenging than usual. Today you'll complete just one double long interval.

Reflect on the Glorious Mysteries today, especially the first Glorious Mystery, The Resurrection and its associated virtue, faith. Do you give witness to your faith or are you ashamed of it? Do you defend your faith to those who criticize it? Are you prepared to do so?

Workout: After the **Cherubim Level Warm-up**, increase intensity to your base pace (RPE of 5-7) and begin praying the Rosary. The double interval begins with the 1st Hail Mary of the 2nd decade and continues until the 10th Hail Mary at the end of the 3rd decade. Recover during the 4th decade, and resume your base pace during the rest of the Rosary. When you finish the Rosary, transition to the **Cherubim Level Cool-down**.

Journal entry: Log your workout in your journal.

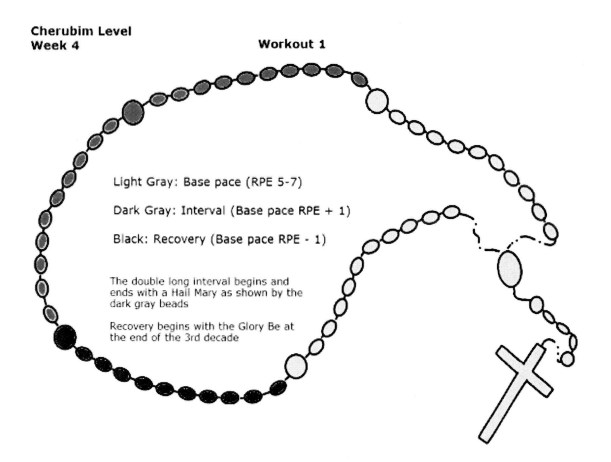

Cherubim Level
Week 4   Workout 1

Light Gray: Base pace (RPE 5-7)

Dark Gray: Interval (Base pace RPE + 1)

Black: Recovery (Base pace RPE - 1)

The double long interval begins and ends with a Hail Mary as shown by the dark gray beads

Recovery begins with the Glory Be at the end of the 3rd decade

Workout 2 – Recovery (30 minutes):

Focus: Invite a friend or family member to accompany you during your workout. You might discuss the Rosary mysteries, the Bible, or your favorite saint. If you can't find a willing partner, then talk to your guardian angel and listen for his guidance today.

Reflect on the Glorious Mysteries today, especially the second Glorious Mystery, The

Ascension and its associated virtue, hope. Do you give in to despair when things look bad? Do you live your life in the hope of eternal life in heaven?

Workout: Following the **Cherubim Level Warm-up** increase intensity to your recovery pace (base pace RPE minus one), and include suggestions for **unstructured time** during a 30-minute workout. If you don't pray the Rosary, reflect on the Ascension and the virtue of hope. Transition to the **Cherubim Level Cool-down** during the last 5 minutes.

Journal entry: Log your workout in your journal.

Workout 3 – Short Intervals (30 minutes total time):

Focus: Since this is a recovery week, decrease the number of short intervals to 4-5 and the duration of your workout to about 30 minutes.

Reflect on the Glorious Mysteries today, especially the third Glorious Mystery, The Descent of the Holy Spirit and its associated virtue, love of God and the gifts of the Holy Spirit. Do you love God with your whole heart, mind and soul? Do you pray to the Holy Spirit and ask Him to bestow His gifts and graces upon you?

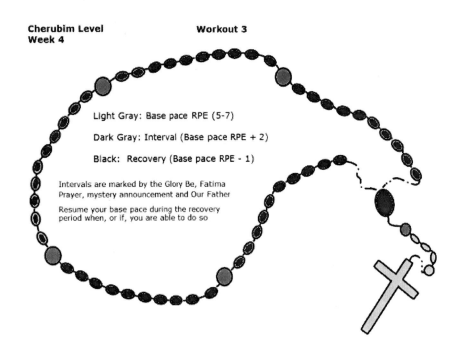

Cherubim Level
Week 4

Workout 3

Light Gray: Base pace RPE (5-7)

Dark Gray: Interval (Base pace RPE + 2)

Black: Recovery (Base pace RPE - 1)

Intervals are marked by the Glory Be, Fatima Prayer, mystery announcement and Our Father

Resume your base pace during the recovery period when, or if, you are able to do so

Workout: After your **Cherubim Level Warm-up**, increase intensity to your base pace (RPE of 5-7) and begin praying the Rosary. Complete 4-5 short intervals at base pace RPE + 2. When you finish the Rosary, transition to the **Cherubim Level Cool-down**.

Journal entry: Log your workout in your journal.

Workout 4 – Base Pace Training (30 minutes total time):

Focus: This workout focuses on base pace training — maintaining your base pace during a 30-minute workout. During the cool-down, think of a good deed that you can do later today.

Reflect on the Glorious Mysteries today, especially the fourth Glorious Mystery, The Assumption and its associated virtue, the grace of a happy death. Are you spiritually prepared for death? If you died today, how would your life be judged?

Workout: Following the **Cherubim Level Warm-up** increase intensity to your recovery pace (base pace RPE minus one), and pray the Rosary during a 30-minute workout. When you finish the Rosary, transition to the **Cherubim Level Cool-down**.

Journal entry: Log your workout in your journal.

Workout 5 – Recovery and Stretching (30-45 minutes total time)

Focus: Reflect on the Glorious Mysteries today, especially the fifth Glorious Mystery, The Coronation (Crowning of Mary as Queen of Heaven and Earth) and its associated virtue, true devotion to Mary. Do you pray for the graces that our Blessed Mother so freely gives to those who ask?

No structured workout today. Instead, warm-up for 10-15 minutes and spend about 15-30 minutes gently stretching. Optional: Include suggestions for **unstructured time**. Be sure to reflect on the fifth Glorious Mystery, the Coronation and its associated virtue, true devotion to Mary.

Journal entry: Log your workout in your journal.

Congratulations! You have completed the Cherubim Level of The Rosary Workout™.

"The Most Holy Virgin in these last times in which we live has given a new efficacy to the recitation of the Rosary to such an extent that there is no problem, no matter how difficult it is, whether temporal or above all spiritual, in the personal life of each one of us, of our families...that cannot be solved by the Rosary. There is no problem, I tell you, no matter how difficult it is, that we cannot resolve by the prayer of the Holy Rosary." - Sister Lucia dos Santos, Fatima seer

Cherubim Level Graduation Requirements

You are ready to move on to the Seraphim Level if you have met the following conditions:

1. You have exercised 5 days each week for 4 continuous weeks.
2. You completed a Rosary Race.
3. You have no symptoms of overtraining.
4. You are familiar with the virtues associated with each of the 20 mysteries of the Rosary.
5a. If you have not met the conditions above, consider extra study and/or workouts before you progress to the Seraphim Level. If you struggle with the workouts, persevere until you are able to meet the goals above. If the intervals are too challenging, perhaps you're not quite ready for this level. Consider repeating the workouts of the Throne Level and then attempt the Cherubim Level workouts at a future date.
5b. Don't get discouraged if you struggle with the spiritual exercises. Keep reflecting on the virtues associated with each mystery and try to gradually incorporate them in your own life.
6. Reward yourself for reaching your goal.
7. Remember to pray to the Choir of Cherubim (and any saints to whom you prayed for intercession) to thank them for their assistance in helping you complete this level.

Cherubim Level Completion Assignments:

<u>For the Soul</u>: Don't forget to go to Confession! If you haven't already, introduce your family to the Rosary. According to Pope John Paul II: *"As a prayer for peace, the Rosary is also, and always has been, a prayer of and for the family. At one time this prayer was particularly dear to Christian families, and it certainly brought them closer together. It is important not to lose this precious inheritance. We need to return to the practice of family prayer and prayer for families." –Rosary of the Virgin Mary*

Even young children can learn the prayers of the Rosary and at least join in a decade. You can play a Rosary CD or tape in your vehicle and pray as a family while you run errands or travel.

If you live alone or if your family members are not Catholic, then contact your parish. Many parishes pray the Rosary as a group. If not, consider starting a Rosary prayer group. Put a notice in the parish bulletin or website, or simply gather a group of friends at a specific time and location to pray the Rosary.

<u>For the Body</u>: If you have not seen a dentist in the past year, it's time for a check-up. Frequent cleanings are good preventative medicine. Some studies show that regular flossing helps prevent heart disease. Good hygiene should include brushing your teeth at least twice a day and flossing at least every other day. Remember to buy a new toothbrush every 3 months.

Seraphim Level Workouts (4 weeks and beyond)

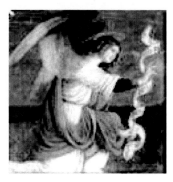

Prayer to the **Choir of Seraphim:**

By the intercession of St. Michael and the celestial Choir of Seraphim may the Lord make us worthy to burn with the fire of perfect charity. Amen.

-From the Chaplet of St. Michael the Archangel

Pray to the Choir of Seraphim and your own guardian angel for assistance in completing this level.

Seraphim Level Summary and Goals:

Congratulations!! You are ready to graduate from the "school" of The Rosary Workout™. You can begin to design your own workout program, using the knowledge and experience you've gained.

Here are the basic principles:

1. Schedule 4-week cycles using the pattern of increasing difficulty until the 3rd (peak) week, followed by a recovery period during Week 4.

2. Change just one or two variables in a given 4-week cycle: **mode, frequency, duration** or **intensity.**

3. Write down the goals you hope to accomplish during the 4-week cycle and plan your workouts accordingly.

4. Alternate your workouts using the Advanced Level cycle -- short interval day, long interval day, recovery day. If you experience overtraining symptoms, take a few days off and analyze what caused you to overtrain before returning to the program, with any appropriate modifications.

5. If you're unsure of how to design the workouts, go back and take a look at the workouts in the intermediate and advanced series. Use them as a foundation and change the frequency, RPE, duration or number of intervals to accommodate your current fitness level.

6. Reward yourself for reaching a goal.

7. Keep your workouts fresh by occasionally trying a new sport or mode of exercise. For example, if you normally ride a mountain bike, try a road bike or take an indoor cycling class.

8. Remember to incorporate prayer into your workouts. In addition to the Rosary, memorize

new prayers, chaplets, litanies, etc. to add to your workouts. The Divine Mercy Chaplet is easy to learn and is a very powerful prayer.

9. Keep up the habit of making a journal entry after each workout.

10. Do a Rosary Race (see Cherubim Level, Week 3 Workout 3) once a month or every 6-8 weeks to track your improvement.

11. Don't forget to go to Confession at least once a month.

12. Work on spiritual growth as well. If you skipped some of the completion assignments for previous levels, then try to incorporate some of the suggestions. Read about devotions to the Sacred Heart, to Mary, or a saint who interests you. Better yet, make an appointment with a priest to ask for guidance on how to enrich your spiritual life.

For more ideas, visit a Catholic bookstore in your area or search online.

"I have competed well; I have finished the race; I have kept the faith." (2 Timothy 4:7)

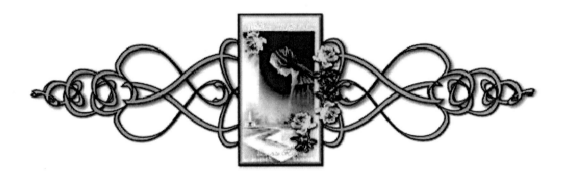

Appendix A: How to Obtain a Rosary in Different Formats

In order to pray the Rosary, you must own or borrow one. If you don't own a Rosary, purchase one online or at a Catholic bookstore or gift shop. Your parish may also sell or give away Rosaries. (Ask a priest to bless your Rosary.) Order a free Rosary at these websites:
http://www.familyrosary.org/main/rosary-rosaries.php
http://www.catholicmissionleaflets.org/form.htm (Postage cost is $1.00)
http://www.rosaryarmy.com (Click "Free Rosary")

Virtual and Audio Rosaries:

Susan Bailey is a singer/songwriter performing prayerful music as an expression of her Catholic faith. She does a number of beautiful and moving songs including her "sung rosary." Visit her website at **www.SungRosary.com.**

The site below allows free downloads of a "virtual" Rosary. The prayers are listed on your computer screen, one line at a time. Your progress through the Rosary beads is graphically illustrated. Although it's not a high-tech program, it is simple and effective.
http://www.virtualrosary.org

Order a free CD on how to pray the Rosary from this site:
http://www.catholicity.com/prayer/rosary.html

Download a free audio Rosary at this site:
http://www.rosaryarmy.com (Click on "Prayers" then "Downloadable Audio Rosaries")

I've found several beautiful Rosary CDs and downloads with background music and/or scriptural passages on both itunes and amazon.com by typing "Rosary" in the search feature:
http://www.amazon.com
http://www.apple.com/itunes/store

If you can get EWTN on your TV or radio, they frequently broadcast the Rosary.

Scriptural Rosaries:

A Scriptural Rosary booklet is very helpful if you're at the beginner level in Mary's school. Such booklets contain verses of Scripture to accompany each Hail Mary. They often include pictures or artwork depicting the mysteries of the Rosary to help focus your meditation with visual cues.

View one online at this site:
http://www.rosaryarmy.com
(Click on "Prayers" then "Scriptural Rosary _____ Mysteries")

Apostle's Creed

I believe in God, the Father Almighty, Creator of Heaven and earth; and in Jesus Christ, His only Son Our Lord, Who was conceived by the Holy Spirit, born of the Virgin Mary, suffered under Pontius Pilate, was crucified, died, and was buried. He descended into Hell; the third day He rose again from the dead; He ascended into Heaven, and sits at the right hand of God, the Father almighty; from thence He shall come to judge the living and the dead. I believe in the Holy Sprit, the holy Catholic Church, the communion of saints, the forgiveness of sins, the resurrection of the body and life everlasting. Amen.

Our Father

Our Father, Who art in heaven, Hallowed be Thy Name. Thy Kingdom come, Thy will be done, on earth as it is in Heaven. Give us this day our daily bread, and forgive us our trespasses, as we forgive those who trespass against us. And lead us not into temptation, but deliver us from evil. Amen.

Hail Mary

Hail Mary, full of grace, the Lord is with thee. Blessed art thou among women, and blessed is the fruit of thy womb, Jesus. Holy Mary, Mother of God, pray for us sinners, now and at the hour of death. Amen.

Glory Be

Glory be to the Father, and to the Son, and to the Holy Spirit. As it was in the beginning, is now, and ever shall be, world without end. Amen.

Fatima Prayer

O my Jesus, forgive us our sins. Save us from the fires of hell. Lead all souls to heaven, especially those in most need of Thy mercy.

Hail Holy Queen

Hail, holy Queen, mother of mercy, our life, our sweetness, and our hope. To thee do we cry, poor banished children of Eve. To thee do we send up our sighs, mourning and weeping in this valley of tears. Turn then, most gracious advocate, thine eyes of mercy toward us, and after this our exile show us the blessed fruit of thy womb, Jesus. O clement, O loving, O sweet Virgin Mary.

(Verse) Pray for us, O Holy Mother of God.
(Response) That we may be made worthy of the promises of Christ.

Note: It is also customary to pray the Litany of Loreto instead of the Hail Holy Queen. The Rosary Workout™ program does not include this litany, but it's a very beautiful prayer that you might include in your Rosary outside the workout program. Many websites and Rosary booklets list the prayers of the litany.

The Rosary Prayer
(Optional prayer at the conclusion of the Rosary)

(Verse) Let us pray:

(Response) O God, whose only begotten Son, by His life, death, and resurrection, has purchased for us the rewards of eternal salvation. Grant, we beseech Thee, that while meditating on these mysteries of the most holy Rosary of the Blessed Virgin Mary, that we may both imitate what they contain and obtain what they promise, through Christ our Lord. Amen.

(Verse) Most Sacred Heart of Jesus,

(Response) Have mercy on us.

(Verse) Immaculate Heart of Mary,

(Response) Pray for us.

There is a traditional "rotation schedule" to help you choose which set of mysteries to meditate upon on a given day:

Monday: Joyful Mysteries
Tuesday: Sorrowful Mysteries
Wednesday: Glorious Mysteries
Thursday: Luminous Mysteries
Friday: Sorrowful Mysteries
Saturday: Joyful Mysteries
Sunday: Glorious Mysteries

The mysteries are usually listed in a timeline order. I've included the virtues, or fruits, along with the Biblical references that describe each event:

Joyful Mysteries:

1. The Annunciation (Humility) Luke 1: 26-38; John 1:14

2. The Visitation (Charity/Love of Neighbor) Luke 1: 39-56

3. The Nativity (Poverty) Luke 2: 6-20; Matthew 1:18-25

4. The Presentation (Obedience) Luke 2: 22-39

5. The Finding of the Child Jesus in the Temple (Joy in finding Jesus; prudence) Luke 2: 41-51

Luminous Mysteries:

1. The Baptism of Jesus (Fidelity to our baptismal promises) Matthew 3:11-17; Luke 3:15-22; John 1:22-34

2. The Wedding Feast at Cana (Faith in Mary's intercession and maternal care) John 2: 1-12

3. The Proclamation of the Kingdom (Conversion of heart) Mark 1:14-15; Matthew 5:1-16; Matthew 6:33; Matthew 7:21

4. The Transfiguration (Desire to become a new person in Christ) Luke 9:28-36; Matthew 17:1-8

5. The Institution of the Eucharist (Love of the Eucharist; active participation at Mass); Matthew 26:26-28; John 6: 33-59

Note: The five Luminous Mysteries, or Mysteries of Light, were introduced in 2002 by Pope

John Paul II in *Rosary of the Virgin Mary*.

Sorrowful Mysteries:

1. The Agony in the Garden (True sorrow for sin; repentance) Matthew 26: 36-46; Mark 14: 32-42; Luke 22: 39-46

2. The Scourging at the Pillar (Modesty and purity; mortification or self-denial) Matthew 27:26; Mark 15:15; John 19:1

3. The Crowning of Thorns (Moral courage; love of our enemies) Matthew 27:29-30; Mark 15:16-20; John 1: 2-3

4. The Carrying of the Cross (Patience, especially when suffering; fortitude) Luke 23: 26-32; Matthew 27:31-32; Mark 15:21; Luke 23: 26-32

5. The Crucifixion (Perseverance; mercy) Luke 23: 33-46; Matthew 27: 33-54; Mark 15: 22-39; Luke 23: 33-47; John 19: 17-37

Glorious Mysteries:

1. The Resurrection (Faith) Matthew 28: 1-10; Mark 16: 1-18; Luke 24: 1-49; John 20:1-29

2. The Ascension (Hope) Mark: 16: 19-20; Luke 24: 50-51; Acts 1: 6-11

3. The Descent of the Holy Spirit (Love of God; gifts of the Holy Spirit) Acts 2: 1-41

4. The Assumption* (Grace of a happy death; eternal happiness) Revelation 12:1

5. The Crowning of Mary as Queen of Heaven and Earth** (True devotion to Mary) Revelation 12:1

* Mary's Assumption and Coronation are implied in Revelation Chapter 12 and in other Biblical references, but neither is directly stated in the Bible. Both events are part of Catholic Tradition. The <u>Catechism of the Catholic Church</u> defines the Assumption in Sections 966 and 974.

**Mary is the "Mother of God," the Queen Mother of Christ the King. Catholics celebrate the feast of the Queenship of Mary annually on August 22nd. Mary is addressed as Queen in many titles that honor her such as Queen of the Rosary, Queen of Peace, Queen of the Angels, etc.

Appendix D: How to Pray the Rosary

A portable music player is a helpful tool for memorization, and I highly recommend this method if you are not familiar with most of the Rosary prayers. There are many Rosary CDs and downloads available. (See Appendix A for resources.)   Listening to an audio version of the Rosary helps you to memorize the prayers and meet the timing goals of the workouts. Obviously, consider any safety issues involved in exercising with headphones. If you don't have access to a portable music player or if safety is an issue, then memorize the prayers before attempting the workouts.

There is a graphic depiction showing how to pray the Rosary at the end of this section. It may be helpful to refer to it while reading the following explanation. The text for each prayer of the Rosary is included in Appendix B. The mysteries of the Rosary are listed in Appendix C.

To pray the Rosary, begin by making the Sign of the Cross (using the Rosary's crucifix held in your right hand) to touch your forehead, chest, left shoulder then right shoulder. Most people hold the crucifix and beads between their thumb and index finger and slide the Rosary to the next bead after each prayer is said in turn.

The first prayer of the Rosary is the Apostles' Creed, a summary of Catholic faith, which uses the crucifix as a marker instead of a bead. Next, move to the first bead on the short chain, which is called the pendant chain. This is a marker for the Our Father. The next three beads, spaced closely together, are markers for three Hail Mary's.

Note: The three Hail Mary beads on the pendant chain are traditionally prayed for an increase in the three theological virtues: Faith, Hope and Charity. The three beads are also said to honor the Three Persons of the Blessed Trinity: Father, Son and Holy Spirit.

After the third Hail Mary bead, there is a longer section of chain between the beads that serves as a cue to pray the Glory Be and Fatima Prayer and to announce the first mystery, which will begin the first decade of the Rosary. To announce the mystery, say (out loud or silently): "The first _____ mystery, _____." (As an example, "The first Joyful Mystery, The Annunciation.")   At this point, you should pause briefly and think about the mystery or recite an appropriate passage from the Bible. This helps to focus your meditation during the upcoming Our Father and ten Hail Mary's. The last bead on the pendant chain is a marker for the Our Father, which is the opening prayer of the first decade.

Note: There are no beads to cue the Glory Be, Fatima Prayer and mystery announcement. The cue is the longer link of chain between the decade of Hail Mary's and the isolated Our Father bead.

Now, move to the circular part of the Rosary. You can go in either direction, skipping the medal that joins the large circular chain to the pendant chain. (The medal prayer is not said until the end of the Rosary.) The ten closely-spaced beads next to the medal (either side) are markers for ten Hail Mary's and are called a decade. A decade marks the time for meditation on the mystery. The repeated Hail Mary's help lull you into a meditative mood through their repetition. They also implore the Blessed Mother to pray for us and to lead us closer to her Son as we reflect on the mysteries of His life, death, Resurrection, and return to heaven.

After the ten Hail Mary beads, there is a longer length of chain that signals the end of your meditation on the first mystery. It also reminds you to pray a Glory Be and the Fatima Prayer and to announce the second mystery (for example, "The second Joyful Mystery, The Visitation"). Remember to pause briefly and visualize or reflect on the upcoming mystery or recite an appropriate Biblical passage to help focus your meditation. The isolated bead (with longer lengths of chain on each side) is a marker for the Our Father. The next ten closely-spaced beads are markers for ten Hail Mary's, which mark the time to meditate on the second mystery.

This pattern continues until the end of the fifth mystery. Pray the Glory Be and Fatima Prayer as usual, but there is no Our Father bead. Instead, pray the Hail Holy Queen using the medal which joins the chains together as a marker. (There is no bead for the Hail Holy Queen.)

Many Catholics add The Rosary Prayer (see Appendix B) and a prayer for the Pope's intentions after praying the Rosary.

Finally, conclude the Rosary by repeating the Sign of the Cross, using the crucifix, as you did in the beginning. Again, some people kiss the crucifix reverently after the Sign of the Cross.

If you would like to review additional references, the links below are helpful tutorials on how to pray the Rosary:
www.erosary.com
www.how-to-pray-the-rosary.com

How to recite the Holy Rosary

1. SAY THESE PRAYERS...

IN THE NAME of the Father, and of the Son, and of the Holy Spirit. Amen. *(As you say this, with your right hand touch your forehead when you say Father, touch your breastbone when you say Son, touch your left shoulder when you say Holy, and touch your right shoulder when you say Spirit.)*

I BELIEVE IN GOD, the Father almighty, Creator of Heaven and earth. And in Jesus Christ, His only Son, our Lord, Who was conceived by the Holy Spirit, born of the Virgin Mary, suffered under Pontius Pilate; was crucified, died, and was buried. He descended into Hell. The third day He rose again from the dead. He ascended into Heaven, and sits at the right hand of God, the Father almighty. He shall come again to judge the living and the dead. I believe in the Holy Spirit, the holy Catholic Church, the communion of saints, the forgiveness of sins, the resurrection of the body, and life everlasting. Amen.

OUR FATHER, Who art in Heaven, hallowed be Thy Name. Thy kingdom come, Thy will be done on earth as it is in Heaven. Give us this day our daily bread, and forgive us our trespasses, as we forgive those who trespass against us. And lead us not into temptation, but deliver us from evil. Amen.

HAIL MARY, full of grace, the Lord is with thee. Blessed art thou among women, and blessed is the fruit of thy womb, Jesus. Holy Mary, Mother of God, pray for us sinners, now and at the hour of our death. Amen.

GLORY BE to the Father, and to the Son, and to the Holy Spirit. As it was in the beginning is now, and ever shall be, world without end. Amen.

O MY JESUS, forgive us our sins, save us from the fires of Hell; lead all souls to Heaven, especially those in most need of Thy mercy. Amen.

HAIL HOLY QUEEN, mother of mercy; our life, our sweetness, and our hope. To thee do we cry, poor banished children of Eve. To thee do we send up our sighs, mourning and weeping in this vale of tears. Turn, then, most gracious advocate, thine eyes of mercy toward us. And after this, our exile, show unto us the blessed fruit of thy womb, Jesus. O clement, O loving, O sweet Virgin Mary. Pray for us, O holy Mother of God, that we may be made worthy of the promises of Christ. Amen.

O GOD, WHOSE only-begotten Son by His life, death and resurrection, has purchased for us the rewards of eternal life; grant, we beseech Thee, that by meditating upon these mysteries of the Most Holy Rosary of the Blessed Virgin Mary, we may imitate what they contain and obtain what they promise, through the same Christ our Lord. Amen.

ANNOUNCE *each mystery by saying something like, "The third Joyful Mystery is the Birth of Our Lord." This is required only when saying the Rosary in a group.*

2. IN THIS ORDER...

INTRODUCTION
1. IN THE NAME...
2. I BELIEVE IN GOD...
3. OUR FATHER...
4. HAIL MARY...
5. HAIL MARY...
6. HAIL MARY...
7. GLORY BE...
8. O MY JESUS...

THE FIRST DECADE
9. ANNOUNCE...
10. OUR FATHER...
11. HAIL MARY...
12. HAIL MARY...
13. HAIL MARY...
14. HAIL MARY...
15. HAIL MARY...
16. HAIL MARY...
17. HAIL MARY...
18. HAIL MARY...
19. HAIL MARY...
20. HAIL MARY...
21. GLORY BE...
22. O MY JESUS...

THE SECOND DECADE
23. ANNOUNCE...
24. OUR FATHER...
25. HAIL MARY...
26. HAIL MARY...
27. HAIL MARY...
28. HAIL MARY...
29. HAIL MARY...
30. HAIL MARY...
31. HAIL MARY...
32. HAIL MARY...
33. HAIL MARY...
34. HAIL MARY...
35. GLORY BE...
36. O MY JESUS...

THE THIRD DECADE
37. ANNOUNCE...
38. OUR FATHER...
39. HAIL MARY...
40. HAIL MARY...
41. HAIL MARY...
42. HAIL MARY...
43. HAIL MARY...
44. HAIL MARY...
45. HAIL MARY...
46. HAIL MARY...
47. HAIL MARY...
48. HAIL MARY...
49. GLORY BE...
50. O MY JESUS...

THE FOURTH DECADE
51. ANNOUNCE...
52. OUR FATHER...
53. HAIL MARY...
54. HAIL MARY...
55. HAIL MARY...
56. HAIL MARY...
57. HAIL MARY...
58. HAIL MARY...
59. HAIL MARY...
60. HAIL MARY...
61. HAIL MARY...
62. HAIL MARY...
63. GLORY BE...
64. O MY JESUS...

THE FIFTH DECADE
65. ANNOUNCE...
66. OUR FATHER...
67. HAIL MARY...
68. HAIL MARY...
69. HAIL MARY...
70. HAIL MARY...
71. HAIL MARY...
72. HAIL MARY...
73. HAIL MARY...
74. HAIL MARY...
75. HAIL MARY...
76. HAIL MARY...
77. GLORY BE...
78. O MY JESUS...

CONCLUSION
79. HAIL HOLY QUEEN...
80. O GOD, WHOSE...
81. IN THE NAME...

3. WHILE TOUCHING THESE BEADS TO KEEP TRACK OF YOUR PROGRESS...

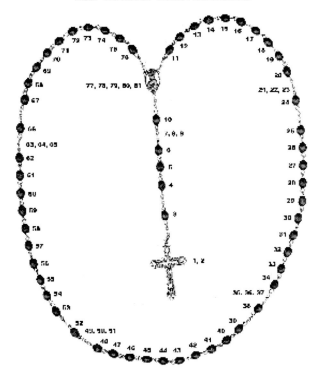

4. AND SILENTLY MEDITATING ON THESE "MYSTERIES", OR EVENTS FROM THE LIVES OF JESUS AND MARY...

On Monday and Saturday, meditate on the "Joyful Mysteries"
First Decade (Steps 9-22): The Annunciation of Gabriel to Mary (Luke 1:26-38)
Second Decade (Steps 23-36): The Visitation of Mary to Elizabeth (Luke 1:39-56)
Third Decade (Steps 37-50): The Birth of Our Lord (Luke 2:1-21)
Fourth Decade (Steps 51-64): The Presentation of Our Lord (Luke 2:22-38)
Fifth Decade (Steps 65-78): The Finding of Our Lord in the Temple (Luke 2:41-52)

On Thursday, meditate on the "Luminous Mysteries"
First Decade: The Baptism of Our Lord in the River Jordan (Matthew 3:13-16)
Second Decade: The Wedding at Cana, when Christ manifested Himself (Jn 2:1-11)
Third Decade: The Proclamation of the Kingdom of God (Mark 1:14-15)
Fourth Decade: The Transfiguration of Our Lord (Matthew 17:1-8)
Fifth Decade: The Last Supper, when Our Lord gave us the Holy Eucharist (Mt 26)

On Tuesday and Friday, meditate on the "Sorrowful Mysteries"
First Decade: The Agony of Our Lord in the Garden (Matthew 26:36-56)
Second Decade: Our Lord is Scourged at the Pillar (Matthew 27:26)
Third Decade: Our Lord is Crowned with Thorns (Matthew 27:27-31)
Fourth Decade: Our Lord Carries the Cross to Calvary (Matthew 27:32)
Fifth Decade: The Crucifixion of Our Lord (Matthew 27:33-56)

On Wednesday and Sunday, meditate on the "Glorious Mysteries"
First Decade: The Glorious Resurrection of Our Lord (John 20:1-29)
Second Decade: The Ascension of Our Lord (Luke 24:36-53)
Third Decade: The Descent of the Holy Spirit at Pentecost (Acts 2:1-41)
Fourth Decade: The Assumption of Mary into Heaven
Fifth Decade: The Coronation of Mary as Queen of Heaven and Earth

www.newadvent.org

Appendix E: Benefits and Blessings of the Rosary

Wouldn't it be wonderful to receive a sign from heaven that you are on the right path? Or to receive heavenly aid, graces and protection in the trials of everyday life? Well those are just a few of the many benefits available to anyone who devoutly and frequently recites the Rosary.

15 Promises of Mary (Given to St. Dominic and Blessed Alan de la Roche):

1. Whoever shall faithfully serve me by the recitation of the Rosary, shall receive signal graces. [Author's note: Signal graces are signs that give us an answer or let us know we are on the right path.]

2. I promise my special protection and the greatest graces to all those who shall recite the Rosary.

3. The Rosary shall be a powerful armor against hell; it will destroy vice, decrease sin, and defeat heresies.

4. It will cause virtue and good works to flourish; it will obtain for souls the abundant mercy of God; it will withdraw the hearts of people from the love of the world and its vanities, and will lift them to the desire of eternal things. Oh, that souls would sanctify themselves by this means.

5. The soul which recommends itself to me by the recitation of the Rosary shall not perish.

6. Whoever shall recite the Rosary devoutly, applying themselves to the consideration of its Sacred Mysteries, shall never be conquered by misfortune. God will not chastise them in His justice, they shall not perish by an unprovided death; if they are just, they shall remain in the grace of God, and become worthy of eternal life.

7. Whoever shall have a true devotion for the Rosary shall not die without the Sacraments of the Church.

8. Those who are faithful to reciting the Rosary shall have during their life and at their death the light of God and the plentitude of His graces; at the moment of death they shall participate in the merits of the Saints in Paradise.

9. I shall deliver from purgatory those who have been devoted to the Rosary.

10. The faithful children of the Rosary shall merit a high degree of glory in Heaven.

11. You shall obtain all you ask of me by the recitation of the Rosary.

12. All those who propagate the Holy Rosary shall be aided by me in their necessities.

13. I have obtained from my Divine Son that all the advocates of the Rosary shall have for

intercessors the entire celestial court during their life and at the hour of death.

14. All who recite the Rosary are my children, and brothers and sisters of my only Son, Jesus Christ.

15. Devotion of my Rosary is a great sign of predestination.

Blessings of the Rosary:

In addition to the many benefits of the Rosary as stated above, there are also abundant blessings for those who devote just 15-20 minutes on a regular basis to this simple but powerful prayer.

1. Sinners are forgiven.
2. Souls that thirst are refreshed.
3. Those who are fettered have their bonds broken.
4. Those who weep find happiness.
5. Those who are tempted find peace.
6. The poor find help.
7. Member of religious orders (priests, nuns and monks) are reformed.
8. Those who are ignorant are instructed.
9. The living learn to overcome pride.
10. The dead (the Holy Souls) have their pains eased by suffrages (prayers of petition).

Benefits of the Praying the Rosary:

1. It gradually gives us a perfect knowledge of Jesus Christ.
2. It purifies our souls, washing away sin.
3. It gives us victory over all our enemies.
4. It makes it easy for us to practice virtue.
5. It sets us on fire with love of Our Lord.
6. It enriches us with graces and merits.
7. It supplies us with what is needed to pay all our debts to God and to our fellow men; and finally, it obtains all kinds of graces for us from Almighty God.

Appendix F: Helpful Tips and Ideas for Exercise

<u>Walking</u> is an excellent mode of exercise, especially for beginners. It requires minimal equipment and can be done just about anywhere in most types of weather. A good pair of comfortable walking shoes is a must. Walk at a brisk pace (like you're late for an important appointment) to get the full benefit of a walking workout. Of course, if you're new to exercise, start slowly and work up to a brisk pace over a few weeks.

<u>For Parents:</u> If you have children, include them. Put the baby in the stroller and older children on bikes, skates, etc. Walk around your neighborhood and say the Rosary out loud or take turns saying the Rosary prayers. This is a great way to help your children stay fit and learn to pray the Rosary. Take your older children to a playground and walk laps around the area while you watch them play. Pray the Rosary as you and your children run through the sprinklers outside on a hot summer day. At the pool, put a young child in an inflatable ring and use it as a kickboard to swim back and forth across the pool, or walk across the pool carrying or pushing a small child in a float. (Obviously, ensure that any other children are under the supervision of a lifeguard or another adult.) Parents of children on sports teams can walk around the sports field or court during practice. <u>Your children's safety is paramount.</u> Modify the workout to ensure that your children are safe.

<u>Exercising at home:</u> No need to buy a gym membership! Of course, you can walk, run, bike, rollerblade, skateboard, etc outside. If circumstances prevent outdoor exercise, there are other options. One is to use an aerobic step/bench to step up and down while praying the Rosary. Look for a step that is adjustable in height so that you can challenge yourself as you improve. Buy, rent or borrow a step aerobics video or DVD to learn some basic moves. Most libraries offer a selection of exercise DVDs and videos, or they may be available through inter-library loan. Check out this great commercial site for a huge selection: **www.collagevideo.com**

Another option for exercising at home is a jump rope, especially for someone who is very fit. It's not the best choice for beginners due to the high impact and quickly elevated heart rate.

A really fun piece of home exercise equipment is a mini trampoline or "Rebounder". If you're a beginner, a senior citizen or are not sure of your balance, purchase one with a detachable hand rail. Try a few moves with the help of a video or DVD. This site sells workout videos and DVDs under the heading of "Rebounder": **www.collagevideo.com**

Yet another option for home exercise is to purchase a piece of equipment such as a treadmill, elliptical trainer, rowing machine, indoor bike, cross-country ski machine, etc. (Tip: Look for these items in the Classifieds in late February/early March. Many people buy exercise equipment in January and never use it.) If you buy used equipment, inspect it carefully. Ask for the owner's manual, or contact the manufacturer if it's not available, to ensure that you set up, use and maintain it correctly. Some owner's manuals can be found online.

At home, make good use of Rosary CDs or tapes to help you keep track of the prayers. If you have cable, EWTN broadcasts the Rosary at various times. Check the schedule on their website: **www.ewtn.com/tv**. EWTN has several different broadcasts of the Rosary so if one doesn't appeal to you, another might. You can record a Rosary program or time your exercise to coincide with the broadcast.

Recommended Websites

Keep in mind that websites do come and go, but the following sites are well-established and very helpful:

Rosary/Catholic sites:

www.rosaryworkout.com
www.sungrosary.com
www.catholicculture.org
www.rosary-center.org
www.catholicmom.com
www.rosaryworkshop.com
www.ewtn.com
www.catholicity.com
www.salvationhistory.com
www.savior.org
www.hail-mary-rosaries.com
www.vatican.va
www.erosary.com
www.how-to-pray-the-rosary.com
www.rosaryarmy.com

Fitness sites:

www.acefitness.org/getfit
www.acsm.org (Click on the link under "Resources" for "General Public")
www.mypyramid.gov
www.mayoclinic.com (Click on "Healthy Living")

Online Catholic bookstores:

www.bezalelbooks.com
www.ignatius.com
www.adoremusbooks.com
www.allcatholicbooks.com
www.sacredheart.catholiccompany.com
www.stgeorgebooks.com

Send an email to contact@rosaryworkout.com for a free copy of the ebook version and to sign up for newsletters and updates to The Rosary Workout.

BIBLIOGRAPHY

Benedict XVI, Supreme Pontiff, "Recitation of the Holy Rosary," May 3, 2008
http://www.vatican.va/holy_father/benedict_xvi/speeches/2008/may/documents/hf_benxvi_spe_20080503_rosary_en.htl

Catechism on the Angels. Detroit: Opus Sanctorum Angelorum, 2006.

Catechism of the Catholic Church. New York: Doubleday, 1994.

De Montfort, Louis. The Secret of the Rosary. Bay Shore, NY: Montfort Publications, 2005.

De Montfort, Louis. True Devotion to the Blessed Virgin. Bay Shore, NY: Montfort Publications, 2006.

EWTN Online. "Chaplet of St. Michael the Archangel." Retrieved May 20, 2008 from Eternal Word Television Network. www.ewtn.com/library/prayer/mikechap.txt

Feeney, Robert. The Catholic Ideal: Exercise and Sports. Arlington, VA: Aquinas Press, 2005.

Feeney, Robert. The Rosary "The Little Summa". Arlington, VA: Aquinas Press, 2003.

Hahn, Scott. Hail Holy Queen. New York: Doubleday, 2001.

John Paul II, Supreme Pontiff. Apostolic Letter, "Rosary of the Virgin Mary," Oct 16, 2002. www.vatican.va/holy_father/john_paul_ii/apost_letters/documents/hf_jpii_apl_20021016_rosarium-virginismariae_en.html

Johnson, Kevin Orlin. Rosary Mysteries, Meditations, and the Telling of the Beads. Dallas: Pangaeus Press, 1996.

Leo XIII, Supreme Pontiff, Papal Encyclical, "On the Confraternity of the Holy Rosary," Sept 12, 1897. www.vatican.va/holy_father/leo_xiii/encyclicals/documents/hf_lxiii_enc_12091897_augustissimae-virginis-mariae_en.html

The Little Manual of the Holy Angels. Detroit: Opus Sanctorum Angelorum, 2006.

McArdle and Katch. Exercise Physiology. Baltimore: Lippincott, Williams and Williams, 2001

New American Bible with Revised New Testament and Revised Psalms. Washington, D.C.: Confraternity of Christian Doctrine, 1991.

Parente, Pascal P. (1998) "Proper Names of the Angels". Retrieved May 19, 2008 from Eternal Word Television Network: www.ewtn.com/library/mary/angel6.htm

The Pieta Prayer Book. Hickory Corners, MI: MLOR Corp., 2006

Pius XI, Supreme Pontiff, Papal Encyclical, "The Increasing Evils," Sept 29, 1937
http://www.vatican.va/holy_father/pius_xi/encyclicals/documents/hf_p-xi_enc_29091937_ingravescentibus-malis_en.html

Pope, H. (1907). Angels. The Catholic Encyclopedia. New York: Robert Appleton Company. Retrieved May 19, 2008 from New Advent: www.newadvent.org/cathen/01476d.htm

Rudden, Dan "A Brief History of the Rosary" from www.erosary.com/rosary/about/history.htm

Saunders, William P. (9/30/04) Choirs of Angels (Part 1), Catholic Herald

A Scriptural Rosary. New Hope, KY: New Hope Publications, 2003.

Shannon, Albert J.M. The Power of the Rosary. Oak Lawn, IL: CMJ Marian Publishers/Soul Assurance Prayer, 1990.

Tilma Full of Rosaries Guild, "Journaling the Bead" Retrieved March 20, 2008 from www.rosaryworkshop.com/HISTORYjournalingBead.htm

Tremeau, Marc. The Mystery of the Rosary. New York: Catholic Book Publishing Co., 1982.

LaVergne, TN USA
07 April 2011
223254LV00003B/151/P